Rapid Assessment: Health Sector Capacity and Response to Gender-based Violence in Pakistan

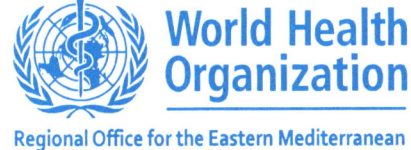
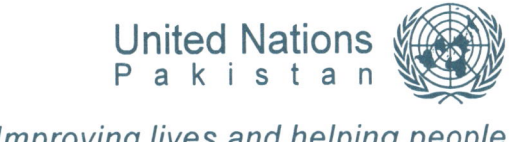
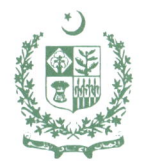

WHO Library Cataloguing in Publication Data

World Health Organization. Regional Office for the Eastern Mediterranean
    Rapid assessment: health sector capacity and response to gender based violence in Pakistan / World Health Organization. Regional Office for the Eastern Mediterranean
    p.
    1. Domestic Violence - prevention & control - Pakistan   2. Battered Women   3. Women's Health   4. Health Care Sector - Pakistan   5. Health Personnel - Pakistan   I. Title   II. Regional Office for the Eastern Mediterranean
    ISBN: 978-92-9021-788-6   (NLM Classification: WA 309.1)
    ISBN: 978-92-9021-789-3 (online)

© **World Health Organization 2011**

All rights reserved.

The designations employed and the presentation of the material in this publication do not imply the expression of any opinion whatsoever on the part of the World Health Organization concerning the legal status of any country, territory, city or area or of its authorities, or concerning the delimitation of its frontiers or boundaries. Dotted lines on maps represent approximate border lines for which there may not yet be full agreement.

The mention of specific companies or of certain manufacturers' products does not imply that they are endorsed or recommended by the World Health Organization in preference to others of a similar nature that are not mentioned. Errors and omissions excepted, the names of proprietary products are distinguished by initial capital letters.

All reasonable precautions have been taken by the World Health Organization to verify the information contained in this publication. However, the published material is being distributed without warranty of any kind, either expressed or implied. The responsibility for the interpretation and use of the material lies with the reader. In no event shall the World Health Organization be liable for damages arising from its use.

Publications of the World Health Organization can be obtained from Health Publications, Production and Dissemination, World Health Organization, Regional Office for the Eastern Mediterranean, P.O. Box 7608, Nasr City, Cairo 11371, Egypt. tel: +202 2670 2535, fax: +202 2765 0424; email: PAM@emro.who.int. Requests for permission to reproduce, in part or in whole, or to translate publications of WHO Regional Office for the Eastern Mediterranean – whether for sale or for non-commercial distribution – should be addressed to WHO Regional Office for the Eastern Mediterranean, at the above address: email: WAP@emro.who.int.

Contents

Acknowledgements	4
Executive summary	5
Chapter 1. Selecting the context	11
Introduction	11
The study	16
Chapter 2. Literature review and analysis	20
Chapter 3. Views and voices of health service providers from the four districts	28
Findings and analysis from the in-depth semi-structured interviews with the health service providers	28
Structured observations by the researcher	53
Chapter 4. Views and voices of women and men from the community from the four districts	56
Findings from the focus group discussions with the men from the community	56
Findings from the focus group discussions with the women from the community	62
Overall impressions from the focus group discussions	69
Chapter 5. Findings and the way forward	73
Findings	73
Policy recommendations for the health sector	81
Specific practical action	83
Annex 1. Interview guide for health service providers in the public sector	87
Annex 2. List of respondents	102
Annex 3. General profiles of the districts included in the study	104
Annex 4. Profiles of the health service providers in the four districts	106
Annex 5. Profiles of the respondents of the focus group discussions	109
References	113

Acknowledgements

This publication is the product of contributions by several individuals. The publication was researched and developed by Dr Rakhshinda Perveen. Technical contributions were also received from Masooma Butt and Dr Ahmed Shadoul, WHO Pakistan and Joanna Vogel, WHO Regional Office for the Eastern Mediterranean.

Executive summary

Global studies have documented that gender-based violence is very common, but that most health care providers fail to diagnose and register it. Often this is due to sociocultural and traditional barriers, lack of time and resources, and inadequate facilities. However, even more so, it is due to lack of awareness and knowledge, poor clinical practice, restricted direct communication and inability to do a full physical examination. In addition, record-keeping is poor with little data on the effectiveness and quality of care. Fear of violence at the household and community level and stigma from society further reduce many victims' willingness to use health services.

The health sector can minimize the prevalence and impact of gender-based violence through improved:

- primary prevention, for example promoting community awareness of prevention;
- secondary prevention, for example early identification, confidentiality, monitoring and respectful treatment of survivors, addressing physical, mental and reproductive health care needs;
- tertiary prevention, for example long-term counselling, mental health care and rehabilitation;
- referral to social, economic and legal support.

Improving the patient–provider interaction is the most feasible, affordable and efficient intervention within any health care system aiming to address the survivors of gender-based violence.

In the structurally and culturally patriarchal society of Pakistan, the public is not sensitized to gender-based violence and the health sector also shares the common societal beliefs and norms, limiting its response to acting only as a public health service provider. Gender-based violence issues are considered "controversial private and domestic issues", not to be taken up as public health problems.

Unfortunately, women are mostly the victims of violence and they face tremendous challenges in disclosing cases of domestic abuse. Even after disclosure, they are met with an unsupportive institutional response and the attitudes of the health providers, medico-legal professionals and law enforcement agencies are often insensitive. Often, the blame is put upon the woman herself. The lack of capacity among health care providers is a key barrier to addressing gender-based violence as a health problem.

WHO Pakistan commissioned a rapid assessment with the primary objective to assess the capacity of the health sector in Pakistan to integrate the issues of gender-based violence. This rapid assessment was conducted under the WHO Gender and Health Programme as part of the One UN Gender Equality Interventions. A qualitative study involving a brief desk review and primary data collection was employed and the total duration of the exercise was 25 days.

Primary data sources included:

- in-depth interviews based on 43 questions that examined different dimensions of the capacities of health service providers of different cadres (medical officers, lady health workers, lady health visitors and executive district officers/district health officers) with 20 such providers, five each in four selected districts (Muzaffarabad district, Azad Jammu and Kashmir; Jamshoro and Hyderabad districts, Sindh; and Kasur district, Punjab);
- eight focus group discussions with men and women who use public sector health facilities;
- consultations with health service providers who participated in a two-day WHO training course on gender-based violence in August 2010 and WHO project officers;
- structured observations by the researcher.

Notwithstanding the biases and limitations attached to the data obtained, the findings of this rapid assessment in the four selected districts will help to plan capacity-building interventions for health care providers to address gender-based violence and give recommendations for gender-based violence protocols and development of standard operating procedures for health delivery staff.

The results contain thought-stimulating findings and challenges and reveal that the health sector has to prepare itself for integrating the complex and sensitive issues of gender-based violence, which are manifestations of existing social inequalities, the brunt of which are borne by women and girls.

The health sector, despite certain strengths such as infrastructure, human resources and renewed political will, is characterized by limited inter-sectoral and multi-sectoral coordination at all levels; poor funding; inefficient utilization of available and allocated health resources and virtually non-existent monitoring and evaluation systems to track progress within the sector in order to make corrective measures. This situation becomes darker when it comes to linking and addressing gender-based violence within the health sectors of Pakistan and Azad Jammu and Kashmir.

The study reconfirms that the connection between gender and health is not only poorly understood but also that gender-based violence is not internalized as a public health issue by the majority of health service providers at different levels.

Critical findings

There is a greater prevalence of gender-based violence and violence against women in its various forms in rural areas. However, the violence faced by urban lower- or middle-class women, including working women and even those within the health sector, also needs to be investigated.

Characteristics of violence include: verbal abuse; physical abuse; hurting emotionally and physically; intimidation; isolation; control over personal things; humiliation; assault; neglect;

threats to children and family; controlling social life, money and food; substance abuse; and taking away liberty and self-expression.

The health sector does not have a policy for addressing gender-based violence. There is no mention of it in the job description of any health service provider and there is no requirement to include it in reporting mechanisms.

The health sector has no data management systems on gender-based violence and has virtually no support mechanisms or inter-sectoral and multi-sectoral links to address the issues of gender-based violence.

The links between disaster management and gender and health are also less understood and visibility cannot be determined.

Health service providers and decision-makers in the health sector are largely driven by the same attitudes, beliefs and laws that are prevalent in all Pakistani society, which discriminate against women in general, and particularly against socially disadvantaged women and men. For instance, although many health service providers shared that they "helped" or "counselled" victims, on probing it was found that "helping" is mostly equated to medical treatment and "counselling" has an emphasis on compromise with the violence or ignoring the crime due to social norms. To a large extent, health service providers are unconvinced of their role in addressing gender-based violence or the relevance of the subject to the health sector.

Health service providers need:

- to understand the relevance of health, gender and gender-based violence;
- to improve their communication skills in relation to gender-based violence;
- to have a clear and consistent understanding of the gender and health needs of different sexes and age groups;
- to clearly understand the social and health outcomes of gender-based violence.

Challenges and conclusions

The key barriers faced by health delivery staff in terms of attitudes and beliefs about violence against women fall into the domains of administrative, technical, community and society.

The perceptions and understanding of health service providers in the public sector at all levels regarding the reasons for, prevalence and characteristics of gender-based violence in their catchment areas, and its impacts on health services, are not very different from the community and society that endorses and legitimizes violence in the name of culture and religion, either under compulsion or by choice.

Gender, if understood at all, is perceived as an entity relating only to women, where there is no role for men who are dominant in their widely infamous role as perpetrators of violence. Integration of gender-based violence into the health sector could lead to a further restriction on the mobility of women and their freedom to visit a health facility imposed by men who control their lives and who would not like any interference by health service providers in this "private matter" (a risk and fear voiced by a lady health worker).

The existing links and capacities (if any) need to be re-examined and strengthened through vigorous and well-coordinated multi-sectoral approaches.

Policy recommendations for the health sector

Integration at policy level

The World Health Assembly, in its 49th Session, declared gender-based violence a global public health emergency. The logical follow-up action is the recognition and integration of gender-based violence as a public health issue into the health policy of each country, articulated loudly and clearly, establishing the political will and readiness of the bureaucratic apparatus to accept, endorse and encourage this integration. Even well-articulated, progressive and inclusive policies in Pakistan fall prey to the problem of ineffective implementation.

The functions of the Federal Ministry of Health are being devolved and provinces will become responsible for, and must develop capacities in, effective health delivery. Integration of gender-based violence issues into provincial health services should preferably be supervised by a female district health officer (currently nearly all are men) at the district level.

Policy-makers must approve guidelines and protocols for standard treatment of women survivors of violence and these must be disseminated not only in English but also in Urdu, Pashto, Sindhi and other local languages at all levels of health care facilities.

Capacity-building of health service providers to address gender-based violence issues

As an important step towards the prevention of gender-based violence, a supportive, violence-aware practice environment should be ensured where health service providers:

- use sympathetic and empowering language appropriate to each patient;
- know how to conduct a physical examination to confirm physical/sexual assault;
- are aware of local services to which abused women can be referred;
- know how to treat not only the physical consequences of abuse but also the mental health ramifications, for example post-traumatic stress disorder.

The abuse of women should be treated as a complicated, multidimensional clinical problem and the provision of specific practical suggestions and resources relevant to the continuum of care, from identification to diagnosis, immediate intervention, and long-term management, should be ensured. To meet such standards, the capacity of the entire administrative machinery and paramedics needs to be built up. This exercise must be preceded by careful research that clearly identifies capacity gaps, training needs and the essential set of information, knowledge and skills to be imparted. Attitudinal and behavioural change exercises must be embedded within such trainings.

Specific practical actions

Training health care providers and raising awareness about gender-based violence will not be enough. Rather, entire health systems need to respond, with links to legal and social services, to support women survivors of violence.

Specific actions include:

- Revamping the medico-legal system, from undergraduate studies to practice, to address weaknesses and make it more professional. An important question is if, and how, alternative measures for meting out justice to sexual assault victims might be prioritized in terms of resource allocation vis-à-vis existing criminal justice and medico-legal practices[1].

- As awareness of existing laws on protection of women from violence is low and their enforcement is half-hearted, an effective dissemination of information on gender-based violence should be ensured through all channels of communication.

- Women's self-help groups and neighbourhood groups could be an effective, socially relevant and sustainable agency to prevent violence.

- Active involvement of key stakeholders, effective players and civil society representatives to develop the ownership on issues of gender-based violence.

- Active involvement of related government line departments at various levels with clear and viable interventions/plans of action for gender-based violence.

- Prompt justice for the victims through establishing the required systems of procedures and coordination.

- Introduction of a survivor-centred approach in programme management within the health sector to address issues of gender-based violence.

Remembering the lesson "addressing gender-based violence calls for a systemic health sector approach", derived from global experiences in improving the response of health sectors to gender-based violence, is one critical step forward.

The need for formative research, exploratory and scoping studies to develop better and clearer understanding of local and indigenous perspectives, issues and priorities on the complex issue of gender-based violence remains of utmost importance.

All recommendations, if considered practically, will contribute towards understanding, new learning and improvements in the health sector and set a standard of recommended practices to address gender-based violence, both in development and in disaster strategies.

---

[1] Borrowed from Du Mont & White (2008), a review commissioned by WHO for the Sexual Violence Research Initiative, an international initiative supported by the Global Forum for Health Research, which is equally valid in Pakistan specific context.

Chapter 1. Selecting the context

Introduction

The United Nations (UN) Declaration on the Elimination of Violence Against Women 1993 defines gender-based violence as:

> "Any act that results in, or is likely to result in, physical, sexual or psychological harm or suffering to women, including threats of such acts, coercion or arbitrary deprivation of liberty, whether occurring in public or in private life".

Gender-based violence, or violence against women,[2] is a major public health and human rights problem throughout the world.

Although violence against women has intense implications for health, it is often ignored. The *World report on violence and health* (WHO, 2002) notes that "one of the most common forms of violence against women is that performed by a husband or male partner". This type of violence is frequently invisible, since it happens behind closed doors. Moreover, legal systems and cultural norms often do not treat it as a crime, but rather as a "private" family matter or a normal part of life. WHO's landmark *Multi-country study on women's health and domestic violence against women* (WHO, 2005)[3] shows that violence against women is widespread, with far-reaching health consequences. It calls on governments to take concerted action and makes recommendations for the health, education and criminal justice sectors to take the problem seriously.

Gender-based violence comes into view as a cause and consequence of gender inequities. It includes a range of violent acts mainly committed by males against females, within the context of women's and girls' subordinate status in society, and often serves to retain this unequal balance (Human Rights Watch, 1996).

Gender-based violence includes, but is not limited to:

- domestic violence by an intrafamily member and intimate partner violence, including physical, sexual or psychological harm, by a current or former partner or spouse;

- sexual violence, including rape, sexual abuse, forced pregnancies and prostitution;

- traditional harmful practices, including female genital mutilation, honour killing and dowry-related violence;

- human trafficking.

---

[2] In this document the terms are used interchangeably.
[3] This groundbreaking research gathered comparable data from over 24 000 women interviewed in 15 sites in 10 countries. The study was implemented by WHO, in collaboration with the London School of Hygiene and Tropical Medicine, PATH, USA, research institutions and women's organizations in the participating countries. The report covers 15 sites and 11 countries: Bangladesh, Brazil, Ethiopia, Japan, Peru, Namibia, Samoa, Serbia and Montenegro, Thailand and the United Republic of Tanzania.

Around the globe, an estimated one in three women will be physically or sexually abused; and one in five will experience rape or attempted rape in their lifetime (BRAC, 2003). Where does most of this violence take place? There is a consensus that gender-based violence takes place in the home, where the victim often experiences repeated attacks. A total of 60%–80% of sexual perpetrators are males known to the victim (Heise, Ellsberg & Gottemoeller, 1999). While men may be exposed to gender-based violence, the health impacts on women are often more. The *Multi-country study on women's health and domestic violence against women* (WHO, 2005), which used a standardized methodology to collect data on intimate partner violence from over 24 000 women from 15 sites in 10 countries, found that:

- the lifetime prevalence of females exposed to intimate partner violence ranged from 20% in Japan, more than 50% in Bangladesh, Ethiopia, Peru and the United Republic of Tanzania, to 70% in Ethiopia; about 15% had experienced intimate partner violence within the past year;
- a total of 4%–32% of all women were exposed to intimate partner violence during pregnancy, ranging from 14% to 32% in low-income countries, compared with 4%–11% in high-income countries;
- about 19% of female adolescents in Mozambique and 48% in the Caribbean had experienced forced sexual initiation.[4]

A large body of evidence documents the often severe and long-lasting impact of gender-based violence on human health including, but not limited to:

- fatal outcomes;
- acute and chronic physical injuries and disabilities;
- serious mental health problems.

Health care providers often serve as the only point of contact with survivors of violence. However, many health care providers fail to diagnose and register gender-based violence. This is not only due to sociocultural and traditional barriers, lack of time, resources and inadequate physical facilities but also due to lack of awareness, knowledge and poor clinical practices with limited direct communication and failure to do a full physical examination or register and monitor the effectiveness and quality of care. Furthermore, the fear of violence and stigma reduces many victims' willingness to use health services (WHO, 1997). Research indicates that a large majority of the victims of violence, usually women and girls, no matter how passive and oppressed, apparently turn to informal networks of friends and community members for help (Heise, Ellsberg & Gottemoeller, 1999). The health sector can minimize the prevalence and impact of gender-based violence through improved:

- primary prevention, for example by promoting community awareness and prevention;

---

[4]Source: *Gender-based violence, health and the role of the health sector* (http://web.worldbank.org/WBSITE/EXTERNAL/TOPICS/EXTHEALTHNUTRITIONANDPOPULATION/EXTPHAAG/0,,contentMDK:22421973~pagePK:64229817~piPK:64229743~theSitePK:672263,00.html, accessed November 2010).

- secondary prevention, for example early identification, confidentiality, monitoring and respectful treatment of survivors, addressing physical, mental and reproductive health care needs;
- tertiary prevention, for example long-term counselling, mental health care and rehabilitation;
- referral to social, economic and legal support.

Improving the patient–provider interaction is the most feasible, affordable and efficient intervention within any health care system aiming to address the survivors of gender-based violence effectively. Many countries are building capacity to prevent and manage gender-based violence and, while the effectiveness of the various approaches still needs to be evaluated, there is no doubt that such violence is preventable.[5]

According to extensive literature reviews documented in the population reports on violence against women (Heise, Ellsberg & Gottemoeller, 1999)[6], it is clear that gender-based violence has implications for almost every aspect of health policy and programming, from primary care to reproductive health programmes (Heise, Ellsberg & Gottemoeller, 1999; Guedes, 2004). Not only do women experience substantial morbidity and mortality as a result of physical and sexual violence, but violence exacerbates other health conditions, including HIV transmission. Increasingly, donors have been addressing violence against women in their health policy and programming portfolios. Indeed, a strategic assessment of the United States Agency for International Development (USAID) global health work revealed that USAID already invests substantial resources in preventing and responding to gender-based violence as a public health issue, albeit in a decentralized way (Bott & Betron, 2005).

Pakistan, with a ranking of 141 on the Human Development Index[7] among 181 countries, a Gender Gap Index[8] of 132 out of 134 countries[9] and with 60.3% of people (with 48% of women in general) living below the poverty line, is struggling with the challenges of gender-based violence. The country is also liable to experience a striking change in socioeconomic development after having being hit by the devastating flood that affected nearly 20 million people and 79 districts.

---

[5] Source: *Gender-based violence, health and the role of the health sector* (http://web.worldbank.org/WBSITE/EXTERNAL/TOPICS/EXTHEALTHNUTRITIONANDPOPULATION/EXTPHAAG/0,,contentMDK:22421973~pagePK:64229817~piPK:64229743~theSitePK:672263,00.html, accessed November 2010).
[6] Source: *Ending violence against women* (http://info.k4health.org/pr/l11edsum.shtml), accessed November 2010.
[7] Latest index according to UNDP (2010) is 125 out of 169 countries.
[8] The *Global gender gap report, 2009* (Hausmann, Tyson & Zahidi, 2009) measures the size of the gender inequality gap in four critical areas:
(1) economic participation and opportunity – outcomes on salaries, participation levels and access to high-skilled employment;
(2) educational attainment – outcomes on access to basic and higher level education;
(3) political empowerment – outcomes on representation in decision-making structures;
(4) health and survival – outcomes on life expectancy and sex ratio.
The Global Gap Index's scores can be interpreted as the percentage of the gap that has been closed between women and men.
[9] Source: *Global gender gap report, 2010* (Hausmann, Tyson & Zahidi, 2010).

Capacity-building[10] is a vital component of any response to gender-based violence in the health sector and needs to be carried out at multiple levels. Also, the type of capacity-building may vary in length, focus and design, depending on the target group and their response to gender-based violence (UNFPA, 2010). Health care workers' basic competencies should include:

- identifying, assessing and documenting abuse;
- intervening to secure safety and reduce vulnerability;
- recognizing that cultural and value factors influence violence against women;
- recognizing legal and ethical issues in intervening and reporting violence against women;
- engaging in activities to prevent violence against women.

In Pakistan, like elsewhere in South Asia, most capacity-building on gender-based violence in the health sector has been training for health service providers, usually in connection with a pilot or project intervention. Pakistan piloted a community-based intervention programme on gender-based violence and HIV in 10 districts, with support from the United Nations Population Fund (UNFPA). This included development of a training module in Urdu and Sindhi and training of more than 300 facility trainers and 240 lady health supervisors. Capacity-building efforts have been facilitated by the development of training manuals and guidelines in a number of countries in the region.

Meanwhile, more long-term, institutionalized capacity-building has been lacking. As in the Pacific and South-East Asia, in Pakistan too, the incorporation of gender-based violence into medical curricula remains a challenge, although Sri Lanka has been successful in integrating a gender-based violence module into its public health orientation training for public health staff who are taking up preventive health positions (medical officers of health) and into the in-service curriculum of public health midwives. Despite concerted effort on the part of many countries, there has been little success in incorporating gender-based violence into medical undergraduate and postgraduate curricula. Reasons for this include lack of prioritization of gender-based violence among academics, a lack of targeted advocacy and a lack of clarity as to which department should be responsible (i.e. forensic, community health, gynaecology, etc.).

WHO Pakistan conducted an analytical report on organizational mapping as part of this rapid assessment to assess gender barriers, particularly in response to issues of gender-based violence in service provision of the health sector in Pakistan. One of the key objectives of this

---

[10] UNFPA (2010) has employed the following definition:
For the purposes of this assessment and report, capacity-building refers to building the capacity of health care providers and other actors in the health sector to respond to gender-based violence in an effective, compassionate and sensitive manner. It includes (but is not limited to): (a) sensitization of ministry of health staff, policy-makers, administrators and community leaders on gender, gender-based violence and appropriate response; (b) sensitization of all health care providers and administrators at an institutional level on gender-based violence as a health issue; (c) training of care providers dealing directly with survivors to identify, provide appropriate care (e.g. injury treatment, counselling and documentation), and offer referral to additional internal and external services (e.g. social work and legal); (d) regular in-service training of care providers to accommodate the rapid turnover of staff; (e) in-depth training on gender-based violence management for leading care providers through study tours, sharing experiences and overseas training; (f) specific training and continuous professional development on relevant gender-based violence policies and protocols to ensure their implementation; and (g) incorporation of gender-based violence training into undergraduate, postgraduate and technical training curricula of care providers.

organizational mapping was to review and analyse the cumulative responses of public and private organizations and institutions countrywide, focusing on issues of gender-based violence pertaining to health in their operations. Secondly, the mapping exercise provided an overview of available potential capacities, the nature of response by health professionals/health care providers and national policy level commitments on this critical health problem. Box 1 summarizes information provided by 17 organizations and institutions all over Pakistan, including Government ministries and projects, UN partner agencies, donors and civil society organizations.

Box 1. Analysis of responses: A mapping of nongovernmental organizations, international nongovernmental organizations and public sector programmes by WHO.

As far as health sector policies are concerned, neither of the Government ministries that deal directly with health and reproductive health (i.e. the Ministry of Health and Ministry of Population Welfare) have exclusive policies, protocols/commitments/standard operating procedures to address gender-based violence. They treat these issues under the guise of "gender equality". National health policy and national population welfare policy do recognize gender equality and services for women's health but are silent, not sensitized, informed but rather reluctant on the issues of gender-based violence while accepting it as a "private or normal routine matter". A similar mentality is evident in the attitudes of health service providers associated with the public sector. However, although the action plans on these policies do refer to issues of gender-based violence, the care services on the ground are focused on referrals and there is no evidence of services and interventions to be implemented on the part of either ministry in the area of gender-based violence.

The Gender Reform Action Plan under the Ministry of Women Development has carried out some work on gender-based violence and health and also has crisis centres and shelter homes for victims. However, one of the key problems is lack of coordination among these three ministries. Although they claim to have common rules of business, in practice they work in isolation.

As far as the private sector is concerned, there are some organizations working on gender-based violence and health issues but the scope of the work is limited to advocacy, sensitization and referral activities. A few organizations, such as the Family Planning Association of Pakistan, also focus on capacity-building of health providers and service delivery. Therefore, the capacities of service providers associated with these types of organizations are improved in terms of screening and recording cases of gender-based violence, psychosocial support and maintenance of privacy.

The capacities of service providers associated with public health facilities may have sensitization on general issues of gender equality through external sources but they do not have the capacity to understand and treat cases of gender-based violence. The health sector requires capacity-building and training on: basic understanding of gender-based violence as a serious health problem; psychosocial support and counselling techniques; and clinical management and treatment of victims of gender-based violence (screening, medical treatment, referral and medico-legal) at all levels, particularly the primary health level. It further requires manuals, guidelines and standard operating procedures focusing on the above-mentioned areas.

Multi-sectoral response is needed to prevent and address gender-based violence, linking it to health problems. The health sector is not able to address this culturally sensitive issue in isolation. The problem of gender-based violence in Pakistan is multifaceted, having social, cultural and legal dimensions. The respondents strongly recommended having a national protocol for the health sector to address gender-based violence in both normal and humanitarian settings, with concrete policy actions to keep national health policy informed with gender issues, particularly gender-based violence.

Recently, the Ministry of Health in Pakistan has shown a very strong commitment for adopting national protocols for gender-based violence in the existing health system. The initiative was a joint venture of One UN in Pakistan and WHO Pakistan.[11] WHO Pakistan therefore decided to undertake a rapid assessment for determining the capacity of the health sector in the country in relation to the complex area of gender-based violence.

The study

Rationale of the rapid assessment

Gender-based violence or violence against women is a serious public health problem and violation of fundamental human rights. In a society such as Pakistan, patriarchal values and structures are culturally deep-rooted and issues of gender-based violence do not have sensitive public recognition. Health sector attitudes are also influenced by these cultural beliefs and norms. Therefore, the health sector response is limited in addressing issues of gender-based violence during the course of public health service provision. Unfortunately, in closed-culture societies, such as Pakistan, gender-based violence is not seriously considered as a public health problem by the health sector but rather acknowledged as a "controversial private and domestic issue".

The unfortunate reality is that mostly women are the victims of violence and they face tremendous challenges in disclosing cases of domestic abuse. Even when women overcome the challenges of disclosure, they meet with an unsupportive institutional response, and the attitudes of the health providers, medico-legal professionals and law enforcement agencies are often insensitive. For example, they may blame the woman and hold her responsible for what has happened to her. The lack of capacity among health care providers is a key barrier to addressing gender-based violence as a health problem.

This 25-day rapid assessment was conducted under the WHO Gender and Health Programme as part of the One UN Gender Equality Interventions. The objectives and suggested list of questions were based on findings of organizational mapping undertaken in the earlier part of 2010, on different services for victims and survivors of gender-based violence. The findings of this rapid assessment in four target programme districts (Muzaffarabad district, Azad Jammu and Kashmir; Jamshoro and Hyderabad districts, Sindh; and Kasur district, Punjab) will help to plan capacity-building interventions for health care providers to address gender-based violence

---

[11] In a three-day workshop (29 September – 1 October 2010) on the health sector response to gender-based violence, organized by WHO under a UN joint initiative towards gender equality, Dr Rasheed Jooma, Federal Secretary Health, in the inaugural session said:
"The health sector can play a very significant role in addressing and assessing gender-based inequalities, discriminations and issues of violence. It is a serious public health problem in health planning, programming and service provision at all level."
"Islam has significantly emphasized equality of gender; we need to understand the values that Islam has laid forward in respecting the gender. Moreover, a health worker has the opportunity to identify and assess gender-based violence. We can incorporate gender education in curriculum of health workers, especially lady health workers/visitors and paramedics so that they can cope with day-to-day gender issues." Source: *The Daily Times* (English), 30 September 2010.

and translate recommendations for protocols and standard operating procedures development for gender-based violence on the response of health delivery staff.

Objectives

The objectives were as follows:

- to assess existing readiness of the health service providers to address gender-based violence in health care service provision in target districts;
- to provide recommendations for improving the capacity of the health sector and its response (i.e. identification, screening, management and recording) to address cases of gender-based violence.

Key areas of enquiry

The key areas of enquiry were:

- key barriers (social, political, administrative, etc.) faced by health delivery staff in terms of attitudes and beliefs about violence against women while providing health services;
- respondents' biases, perceptions and understanding of reasons, prevalence and characteristics of gender-based violence (i.e. physical, psychological and sexual abuse from in-laws, other relatives, colleagues, etc.) in their catchment areas, as well as its perceived impact on health;
- respondents' existing capacity to identify hidden symptoms of gender-based violence and whether they referred survivors to local psychosocial services;
- support mechanisms and existing resources for health care providers/delivery staff to address cases of gender-based violence, including the presence of female health care providers;
- existing health sector capacities and links with other sectors/line departments/civil society organizations to address gender-based violence, including identifying gender-based violence, sensitive ways of communicating with patients (i.e. capacity to engage victims in conversation), responding to and documenting cases of gender-based violence;
- health sector structural readiness to address gender-based violence:
  - levels of privacy in health centres, effective sound and visual barriers;
  - how medical records are stored and who has access to them;
  - capacity to maintain privacy and confidentiality;
  - referral to, and awareness of, available resources/support (medical care, medico-legal information);

- capacity and resources available for consistent recording of cases of gender-based violence.

Methods

A qualitative research study was designed to conduct this rapid assessment. Data sources included primary and secondary sources.

Samples and primary data collection sources were:

- Twenty semi-structured in-depth interviews with five levels of health service providers (lady health visitors, lady health workers, medical officers (male and female), executive district officers, health/district health officers or medical superintendents) from each district were conducted. The number of health service providers was purposive but their selection was at random.
- Eight focus group discussions with consumers of health services, i.e. community members, were conducted in all four selected districts. Two focus group discussions with users of the public sector health services, one with men and another with women, were organized in each district and the process was coordinated by a credible local voluntary organization. Each focus group discussion consisted of a minimum of five and a maximum of eight participants. The numbers of focus group discussions and respondents were purposively decided but the local facilitator in each district randomly selected the individuals.
- Consultations: three group discussions were held (one in Sindh for Jamshoro/Dadu/Hyderabad-based participants; one in Sindh; one in Muzaffarabad, Azad Jammu and Kashmir; and one in Kasur, Punjab) with health service providers who attended the two-day training on gender organized by WHO Pakistan in August 2010. In addition, telephone, face-to-face and e-mail consultations were conducted with some project officers and WHO Pakistan programme managers and experts in public health to validate certain findings and ascertain organizational mandates and institutional mechanisms.

Data collection instruments (questionnaires) for each category of respondents and a guide are attached in Annex 1. The tools for the semi-structured interviews were pretested in Islamabad with local health service providers and changes were made accordingly. Data were then collected using English and Urdu versions in the districts. Informed consent was provided by all respondents.

Field observations by the researcher were also employed as a source of primary information. Besides random observations made while interpreting and analysing the qualitative information, a structured set of observations was also made in conformity with the instrument given in Annex 1.

Secondary data collection included a brief desk review and analysis of published material, mostly available on the World Wide Web, regarding gender-based violence and its integration into the health sector in the past 10–15 years. It also assembled lessons learnt from global, including South Asian, experiences in the citizen sector and public policies.

Limitations and biases (sampling biases, time constraints, language limitations and biases) of the methodology were identified in advance and the results have been interpreted accordingly.

The study did not focus on specific health issues related to gender-based violence, such as HIV and AIDS. Furthermore, the study did not accurately and precisely determine the level of knowledge of the health service providers regarding clinical management of sexual violence, and gender-based violence and medico-legal procedures. The study also did not examine the political and economic contexts of Pakistan and Azad Jammu and Kashmir. Quality assurance and research ethics have been ensured at each and every stage of the research study.

It is also emphasized that, while every effort has been made to gather all relevant information from many stakeholders, this has been predominantly a rapid assessment conducted within a limited time frame. Therefore, the information contained in the report may have certain gaps as valid for all qualitative studies with small samples and the results should not by any means be generalized for the entire population.

A list of the respondents and coordinators involved in the study is attached as Annex 2, while profiles of the four districts are given in Annex 3.

Chapter 2. Literature review and analysis

A global literature review was conducted as an initial step for collating essential information and evidence on gender-based violence as a public health issue.

Most of the reference material was searched on the World Wide Web. The key words used to find the material included: gender-based violence; health sector response to gender-based violence or violence against women; capacity of health sector to integrate gender-based violence or violence against women; and gender and health. The references included in this desk review have been published in the past 10–15 years and although the intention was to use only the most recent literature, older material was used where there was no alternative.

The national literature review gives a snapshot of the health sector and systems in Pakistan and the issues surrounding gender-based violence.

Global literature review

Both non-abused and abused women visit health facilities but what is consistent from the research is the more frequent visits of women who are experiencing violence of any form.[12]

According to worldwide research, the only institution that connects with almost every woman at some point in her life is the health care system. Health service providers, especially those serving in accident and emergency wards and in women's health settings such as sexual and reproductive health, maternal child health and prenatal settings, have a critical role to play in detecting, referring and caring for women living with violence. Interventions by health service providers can potentially mitigate both the short- and long-term health effects of gender-based violence against women and their families.[13] While assessing the health sector response to gender-based violence in the specific context of the Asia Pacific region, a very important and critical point is the vital need to remember that the health system in any country is "not immune" from gender-based violence internally (UNFPA, 2010).[14]

---

[12] Although men can also be victims of intimate partner and sexual violence, this type of violence affects women disproportionately. For instance, both males and females report sexual coercion, but the majority of victims are female and the vast majority of perpetrators are male (USAID, 2008).

[13] "Experience has shown that public health approaches to violence can make a difference. The health sector has the unique potential to deal with violence against women, particularly through reproductive health services, which most women will access at some point in their lives." Source: Joy Phumaphi, Vice President, Human Development Network, World Bank, formerly, Assistant Director General, General, Family, and Community Health, WHO (http://www.who.int/gender/violence/who_multicountry_study/summary_report/chapter1/en/index2.html, accessed November 2010).

[14] UNFPA has highlighted that reproductive rights violations in the health sector (such as unavailability or disruption of contraceptive supplies, judgmental or biased treatment based on reproductive status or choice, coercive family planning counselling, denial of contraceptives and forced sterilization) are forms of gender-based

Box 2. Categories of domestic violence (UNFPA, 2001).

- *Abuse* is a pattern of physical assaults and threats used to control another person. It includes punching, hitting, choking, biting, throwing objects at a person, kicking and pushing and using a weapon such as a gun or a knife.
- *Physical abuse* usually escalates over time and may end in the woman's death.
- *Sexual abuse* is the mistreatment or the control of a partner sexually. This can include demands for sex using coercion or the performance of certain sexual acts, forcing her to have sex with other people, treating her in a sexually derogatory manner or insisting on unsafe sex.
- *Emotional and verbal abuse* is the mistreatment and undermining of a partner's self-worth. It can include criticism, threats, insults, belittling comments and manipulation on the part of the batterer.
- *Psychological abuse* is the use of various tactics to isolate and undermine a partner's self-esteem, causing her to be more dependent on, and frightened of, the batterer. It can include such acts as:
  - refusing to allow the woman to work outside the home;
  - withholding money or access to money;
  - isolating her from family and friends;
  - threatening to harm people and things she loves;
  - constantly checking up on her.

Box 2 lists the different categories of domestic violence. The short-term, immediate and long-term effects of different forms of violence in the lives of women and girls are an amalgam of a wide range of physical, mental and reproductive health consequences, which often last long after the abuse has ended (Garcia-Moreno et al., 2005). The research is conspicuous by the lack of effort in exploring links between gender-based violence and infectious diseases, apart from sexually transmitted infections such as HIV.[15] The most common fatal health outcomes of gender-based violence are homicide and suicide; other outcomes with huge social disadvantages include sexually transmitted infections, including HIV. An effective response to these outcomes can only be initiated if ample research is available in these areas (USAID, 2008).

In a report on violence against women and girls (WHO, 2002), key health consequences of gender-based violence are documented as follows:

- Physical:
  - abdominal/thoracic injuries;
  - bruises and welts;
  - lacerations and abrasions;
  - fractures and breaks;
  - eye injuries;

---

violence. This should be considered when undertaking institutional capacity-building related to gender-based violence.

[15] Qualitative research shows that the intersections of HIV, gender inequality and gender-based violence lie in the patriarchal nature of most societies, especially in ideals of masculinity that are predicated on control of women and valorize male strength and toughness (Jewkes & Morrell, 2010).

- o rupture of the eardrum;
- o burns;
- o chronic pain syndromes;
- o disability;
- o gastrointestinal disorders;
- o fibromyalgia;
- o reduced physical functioning.

- Sexual and reproductive:
    - o gynaecological disorders;
    - o pregnancy complications;
    - o miscarriage/low birth weight;
    - o pelvic inflammatory disease;
    - o sexual dysfunction;
    - o sexually transmitted infections, including HIV/AIDS;
    - o unsafe abortion;
    - o unwanted pregnancy.

- Psychological and behavioural:
    - o alcohol and drug abuse;
    - o depression and anxiety;
    - o eating and sleep disorders;
    - o feelings of shame and guilt;
    - o phobias and panic disorders;
    - o physical inactivity;
    - o poor self-esteem;
    - o post-traumatic stress disorder;
    - o psychosomatic disorders;
    - o smoking;
    - o suicidal behaviour and self-harm;
    - o unsafe sexual behaviour.

- Fatal health consequences:
    - o AIDS-related mortality;
    - o maternal mortality;
    - o homicide;
    - o suicide.

The following possible signs[16] of domestic abuse have been documented in a handbook published by the Department of Health, United Kingdom of Great Britain and Northern Ireland (DoH, 2005):

- frequent appointments for vague symptoms;
- injuries inconsistent with explanation of cause;
- woman tries to hide injuries or minimize their extent;
- partner always attends unnecessarily;
- suicide attempts – particularly with Asian women;
- history of repeated miscarriages, terminations, stillbirths or preterm labour;
- repeat presentation with depression, anxiety, self-harm or psychosomatic symptoms;
- non-compliance with treatment;
- frequent missed appointments;
- multiple injuries at different stages of healing;
- patient appears frightened, overly anxious or depressed;
- woman is submissive or afraid/reluctant to speak in front of her partner;
- partner is aggressive or dominant, talks for a woman or refuses to leave the room;
- poor or non-attendance at antenatal clinics;
- injuries to the breasts or abdomen;
- recurring sexually transmitted infections or urinary tract infections;
- early self-discharge from hospital.
- South Asia[17] and gender-based violence

South Asia consists of seven countries (Afghanistan being a recent addition, making eight) and is characterized by its dense population, political conflicts and patriarchy.[18] A mushrooming nongovernmental organization sector and a vibrant women's movement towards gender equality are yet to shake patriarchal structures, and patriarchal values remain deeply ingrained across the dissimilar and unequal communities of South Asia (UNFPA, 2010).

---

[16] None of the above signs automatically indicates domestic abuse but they should raise suspicion and prompt the health service provider to make every attempt to see the woman alone and in private to ask her if she is being abused. Even if she chooses not to disclose at this time, she will know that the providers are aware of the issues and she may choose to approach them at a later time.

[17] There are seven countries, including Pakistan, but not each country is focused on evenly. Selected cases are highlighted.

[18] South Asia is home to 1.7 billion people, well over one-fifth of the world's population, making it both the most populous and most densely populated region in the world. It is also home to nearly half of the world's poor, has the highest illiteracy rate in the world and the schooling of females still lags behind that of males, despite the economic progress that has taken place in some countries. In addition, one-third of the world's maternal deaths occur in South Asia (UNFPA, 2010).

Harmful traditions and practices, such as female foeticide, female infanticide, child marriages, dowry and related abuses and honour killings are tolerated in the name of culture or religion and are either ignored by law-enforcing agencies or never brought under any court due to non-existent, deficient or discriminatory laws and legislations.

UNFPA (2010) has noted that the practices of antenatal sex selection and female infanticide are still prevalent in South Asian countries. Furthermore, many children suffer from malnutrition, with girls being disproportionally affected. The issue of dowry continues to play a role in global-based violence in the region, despite anti-dowry laws enacted in countries such as Bangladesh, India and Pakistan. Disputes about dowry in parts of South Asia have been highlighted as galvanizing serious incidents of domestic violence, including murder and suicide.

Some forms of violence that enjoy legitimacy from society at large are complex to explain. It is difficult to understand the concept that honour lies in a woman's body and men in society are allowed to monitor this honour and display their control in the form of anger, physical and mental abuse, trading and even killing.

Within this cultural context, domestic violence still remains the most prevalent form of gender-based violence. A study from Maharashtra, India, showed that 38% of women were verbally abused and more than half of these had experienced physical abuse by an intimate partner (UNFPA, 2010).

In Bhutan, a study commissioned by the National Commission of Women showed that violence is prevalent in most women's lives, whether they are married or single. It also indicated that alcohol and financial matters were common triggering factors (UNFPA, 2010).

One of the higher prevalence rates of violence against women was reported in Nepal where 80% of women reported psychological violence, 32% reported physical violence and 10% reported sexual violence (UNFPA, 2010).

In Sri Lanka, there are no national guidelines for gender-based violence but national guidelines on management of rape victims are being developed with the assistance of the College of Forensic Pathologists of Sri Lanka and others. A proposal to develop national guidelines for the management of victims of gender-based violence, targeting medical officers, has been accepted by the National Committee on Violence (UNFPA, 2010).

Bangladesh has developed a comprehensive protocol for the Women Friendly Hospitals Initiative, with gender-based violence as one of the four areas of the initiative (UNFPA, 2010).

The Indian Medical Association, in collaboration with United Nations Children's Fund (UNICEF) and the Ministry of Human Resource Development, has developed an examination kit for victims of sexual abuse (UNFPA, 2010).

Guiding principles

> "As is the case for family planning, maternal health, and HIV services, work in the area of gender-based violence requires careful attention to confidentiality, privacy, informed consent, and issues of disclosure. Given the potential risks to survivors, existing data on 'good practice' in this field suggest that organizations should follow some basic

principles when designing and implementing gender-based violence activities. Overall, the principle of 'doing no harm' should guide every decision made." (USAID, 2008)

More specific principles included in the USAID (2008) guide are:

- ensure that all activities respect survivors' safety and autonomy first and foremost ;
- ensure the relevance and appropriateness of interventions to the local setting;
- employ both a public health and a human rights perspective;
- encourage multisectoral interventions at multiple levels;
- invest in evaluation both for the sake of assessing results and for protecting survivors' safety.

Regarding national protocols on gender-based violence, UNFPA (2010) recommends that these must be:

- developed through extensive consultation and consensus-building with stakeholders such as forensic pathologists, gynaecologists, police and social welfare organizations so that there is widespread acceptance of the tool;
- developed at national level and accompanied by a directive from the health ministry to ensure implementation;
- user-friendly to ensure implementation;
- accompanied by a guidance document or training for all relevant hospital departments (including paediatrics, obstetrics/gynaecology, laboratory, emergency, etc.);
- made easily accessible and available in the workplace.

Evidence from studies suggests that rates of gender-based violence are highest in settings where social norms support gender inequality, where communities fail to punish men who use physical or sexual violence against women, and where violence against women is considered normal.[19]

Prevention of violence and protection require careful calculation of the merits and demerits of each strategy and focus. The community can either prevent or perpetuate violence. From a public health perspective, community-level risk factors may be used for recognizing better ways to reduce, if not eliminate, violence against women. Focusing too much on individual risk factors may obscure the fact that "violence against women tends to occur throughout society and across all demographic and socioeconomic groups and appears to be heavily influenced by community norms and responses" (USAID, 2008).

A global review[20] by Du Mont & White (2007) summarized the following lessons from the literature. Sociocultural contexts characterized by male dominance, anti-woman biases and

---

[19] "Do not allow 'culture' or 'tradition' to be used to justify gender-based violence; reframe the issue as a public health problem and a human rights violation" (USAID, 2008, p.12).
[20] Commissioned by WHO for the Sexual Violence Research Initiative, an international initiative supported by the Global Forum for Health Research.

rape-supportive attitudes present a number of barriers to the effective use of medico-legal evidence. In these (and other) contexts:

- The collection of viable medico-legal evidence requires:
    - easily accessible, cost-free (to the victim) male and female sexual assault examiners who are well trained and authorized to gather evidence properly and testify to it in court, and who are sensitized to the negative impacts of erroneous beliefs and attitudes regarding sexual assault and sexually assaulted women;
    - suitable facilities distributed across urban and rural areas, available 24 hours a day, seven days a week, that house adequate supplies and equipment and that can secure the protection of the medico-legal evidence;
    - collaborative networks and effective communication across the health care, law enforcement and legal sectors, and nongovernmental and community organizations such as rape crisis centres;
    - well-constructed standardized protocols adaptable to local circumstances and suitable technologies that are readily available.

- Processing of viable medico-legal evidence requires:
    - access to forensic facilities with adequate resources, staffed by properly trained analysts who can both process the evidence and testify to it without the interference of personal biases and demands from other post-sexual assault professionals;
    - proactive involvement of police specially trained to maintain the chain of custody and to handle cases in a timely and sensitive manner, free from anti-woman, rape-supportive beliefs and attitudes, and corruption;
    - prosecutors, defence attorneys, judges and other court staff sensitized to the detrimental impact that anti-woman biases and rape myths can have on its use in the courts.

The assessment by UNFPA (2010) for its Asia Pacific Region shows that the majority of countries in that Region are actively seeking to respond to the issue of violence. Most countries have initiated or are initiating at least some health sector responses to global-based violence, which is promising. However, there is understandably a wide variation in the scale, scope, quantity and quality of the responses across countries and the level of integration that has been achieved in each country's national health system. Some countries have been addressing gender-based violence through the health sector for more than 10 years (e.g. Indonesia, Malaysia) and have therefore had some success in "scaling-up" pilot projects to integrate a response to gender-based violence into their national health system. Other countries are just starting interventions (e.g. China, Mongolia) and focusing on one particular area, such as capacity-building of health service providers or carrying out pilot projects in a small number of regions and learning lessons for the next steps.

Gender-based violence is a public health issue; however, recognizing this must not imply that the health sector can be expected to deal with it alone. What is important for decision-makers is to understand the technical necessity of a concerted and coordinated effort from a range of sectors, including social services, religious organizations, the judiciary, police, media and business, to reduce and respond adequately to gender-based violence. The health sector therefore needs to play an important role within a multisectoral framework.[21]

---

[21] Violence against women also severely constrains development, obstructing women's participation in political, social and economic life. The impacts include escalating costs in health care, social services and policing, and an increased strain on the justice system. It lowers the overall educational attainment and mobility of victims/survivors, their children and even the perpetrators of such violence. Violence against women undermines and constrains the achievement of the Millennium Development Goals, including those set in the areas of poverty, education, child health, maternal mortality, HIV/AIDS and overall sustainable development. Sources: UN, 2006; Commonwealth of Australia, 2008; UNFPA, 2010.

Chapter 3. Views and voices of health service providers from the four districts

"Yay to roz ka mamool hay kabhi husband biwi ko marta hay to kabhi bhai ya bap marta hay to un ko hum hi treatment kartay hain." (This is the daily routine, sometimes the husband beats the wife and sometimes the brother or father beats her and then we offer them (women) the treatment.) (A lady health worker from Sindh province, Pakistan, 3 November 2010)

This chapter presents the findings of the rapid assessment of the health sector's readiness to integrate gender-based violence in Pakistan, including Azad Jammu and Kashmir, based on data collected through field interviews, discussions and observations in the selected four districts (see methodology in Chapter 1).

This chapter presents the key findings and analysis, district-wise, drawn from and embedded within the responses of the selected respondents. For a clear understanding of the discussion and analysis in this assessment, readers may refer to the brief definition of each concept given in the glossary.

As mentioned while describing the methodology, this assessment is aimed in particular at the viewpoints of lady health workers, lady health visitors, male and female doctors and health officers (executive district officers/district health officers) at the district level. However, it is important to recognize that this by no means is an assessment of the performance of a particular health facility and of any health service provider. Hence, the specific identities of all health facilities have been withheld in the public copy of the report and the same has been observed for the health service providers (lady health visitors, lady health workers and medical officers) who did not give consent to include their names in the list of respondents. The narrative and analytical version of the interviews with the executive district officers/district health officers is also not given, as in so doing their specific identities would be disclosed. These considerations are in conformity with the ethics that must be observed in a research study on a sensitive issue such as gender-based violence and with public sector employees.

It is important to remain cognizant that the responses of those included in the study may not necessarily represent all stakeholders within the health sector in the particular context of gender-based violence but rather these findings attempt to highlight the key trends.

Findings and analysis from the in-depth semi-structured interviews with the health service providers

For each district, an account of each health service provider's interview is given in a synthesized form. Some selected quotes from the interviews are added to establish a direct contact between reader and respondent. The responses of all health service providers are based on the 20 questions extracted from the data collection instrument (see Table 2).

> *"Yay to aam bat hay k Pakistan mein aurtoon ko paon ki joti samjha jata hay par ab ja kay kuch media nay logon ki ankhein kholi hain."* (It is a matter of common perception that women are equated to a footwear but now the media to a certain extent has opened the eyes of the people.) (Response from a lady health worker from Sindh province, Pakistan, 3 November 2010)

Most of the health service providers had heard of the word "gender". However, most could not differentiate between the terms "sex" and "gender" at the conceptual level. Among lady health visitors and lady health workers, those who attended a health session in connection with a family and reproductive health programme, or those who had attended the two-day workshop organized by WHO in 2010, understood the word gender (*sinf*). It should be noted that Table 4 in Annex 4 needs to be carefully evaluated and understood as one could be misled by seeing all "Yes" as response. Nearly all health service providers who were interviewed were familiar with the word (in English and in Urdu language) but were not familiar with the jargon "gender-based violence" or "violence against women, girls and children". An exploration by the interviewer discovered that all health service providers were well aware of all forms of violence. An in-depth session further clarified the exact level of understanding and perception, while also disclosing biases. Some knew that it was "nice and wise" to admit that gender-based violence is a public health issue but "in fact there is no such relation" or "what can health service providers do about violence against women"? Therefore, for all practical purposes, policy-makers and donors should aim to integrate gender-based violence into the health sector at a beginner's level.

There was general agreement that women face different forms of violence in their lives but there was also a reluctance to admit or accept that any form of violence happens in their vicinity. It was encouraging to note that, following rapport-building, the same respondents opened up and, without refuting the earlier answer, discussed in detail different forms of violence. Nearly all the respondents talked about psychological and socially induced forms of violence other than the more overt forms that may or may not require medico-legal action. However, doctors felt more comfortable dealing with physical forms of violence as this is where they saw their perceived relevant role, for example treating physical ailments or wounds, but if the same gender-based violence involved medico-legal action, they were uncomfortable because they knew the convoluted pathways in the medico-legal system only too well.

The most frequent reasons cited as the root causes of gender-based violence included poverty, preference for a son and lack of education. The most common expressions of violence against women, girls and children were nutritional discrimination, sex-selective abortion, and abuses in the customs and institutions of marriage and dowry.[22] Other common forms of violence included wife battering, acid burns, attempted suicide due to mental stress, homicides (honour killing), rape and gang rape. However, most respondents could not justify how poverty encouraged a man to beat his wife, as opposed to a male friend or relative. Some health service providers thought that education could not stop a man from violent behaviour or abuse, therefore emphasis must be on changing this mindset through effective public awareness campaigns at the community level through popular media. Lady health visitors and lady health

---

[22] Only one respondent in Sindh said that dowry was not an issue.

workers were relatively unreserved when talking about the violence against women and girls that was being committed nearly round the clock but they were careful not to give details or disclose names.[23]

Table 1 summarizes the training status of the health service providers. The knowledge and training status of the 20 health service providers in each district is given in Tables 1–4 in Annex 4.

Table 1. Training status of the 20 health service providers included in the study.

Health service provider (no. of respondents)	No. of respondents who received training on gender	No. of respondents who received training on gender-based violence	No. of respondents who received training on gender and health issues	No. of respondents who received training on health issues
Lady health workers (4)	1/4	1/4	1/4	4/4
Lady health visitors (4)	0/4	0/4	1/4	4/4
Male medical doctor (4)	2/4	0/4	2/4	4/4
Female medical doctors (4)	2/4	1/4	3/4	4/4
Executive district officer/district health officer (4)	0/4	0/4	1/4	4/4
Total out of 20 (from each district)	5/20	2/20	8/20	20/20

Hyderabad district, Sindh

Key findings from the female doctor's interview[24]

Gender-based violence and health-related considerations

The respondent was of the view that a female medical doctor could, at least to a certain extent, offer assistance to a victim of violence. She believed that the root cause of gender-based violence lay in the economy and the rising incidence of mental stress. In her opinion, menstrual hygiene, pregnancy, emotional stress and poor nutrition affect a woman's health at different stages of her life. She believed that expectant mothers are granted the opportunity to visit any health facility when they are too unwell or unable to do household chores.

---

[23] This underscores the need and relevance of strongly enforced laws against gender-based violence as these are also helpful for the victims and also serve as a deterrent to the practices of gender-based violence (observation by the WHO review team).
[24] Interviewed on 5 November 2010.

> *"Jab laachaar ho jatee hain tab clinic lai jatee hain."* (When a woman is really helpless then she is brought here – to any health facility.)

In her opinion, gender-based violence affects not only the health of the woman but also influences the health and happiness of her children.

Reported gender-based violence related experience

The respondent had a vast experience of dealing with the medico-legal cases of sexual assault and rape of minor girls and adult women. However, she was not happy with her experience of court appearances, as she found the lawyers' behaviour and choice of words very gender insensitive and culturally inappropriate.

Integration of services for gender-based violence

The female doctor thought that integration of services for gender-based violence at the primary care level, and especially in antenatal care clinics, can only be successful if health professionals are specially trained for this and have counselling skills. In her opinion, the health facility is not currently equipped to address issues of conjugal or domestic violence.

Gender-based violence, the health sector and the post-flood scenario

The respondent was of the opinion that violence against women has increased due to the increased stress caused by the flood damage. She had doubts regarding the health sector's preparedness to address the needs of half a million flood-affected pregnant women and patients and clients from various age groups, but also said that certain health facilities with good staff could manage the increased case-load.

Gender-based violence and the medico-legal system

Doctors carry out medico-legal procedures in cases of rape and sexual assault in the light of the Hudood Ordinance[25]; however, the respondent thought that this is, itself, an instrument of violence as it is a gender-insensitive and discriminatory law. She had no knowledge of any other laws or policies relating to violence against women. When the researcher tried to seek the respondent's views on the said ordinance, she replied "no comment".

Key findings from the male doctor's interview[26]

Gender-based violence and health-related considerations

> *"Syed larki tou bahir ja hee nahi sakti."* (Girls belonging to Syed families are not allowed to marry outside their families/or a non-Syed man is never considered eligible for them.)

---

[25] The Hudood Ordinance (also spelled Hudud) was a law in Pakistan that was enacted in 1979 as part of then military ruler Zia-ul-Haq's Islamization process and replaced/revised in 2006 by the Women's Protection Bill. The Hudood law was intended to implement Islamic Sharia law, by enforcing punishments mentioned in the Quran and Sunnah for Zina (extramarital sex), Gazf (false accusation of Zina), Offence Against Property (theft), and Prohibition (the drinking of alcohol). The ordinance has been criticized as leading to "hundreds of incidents where a woman subjected to rape, or even gang rape, was eventually accused of Zina and incarcerated", and defended as punishment ordained by God and victim of "extremely unjust propaganda".

[26] Interviewed on 5 November 2010.

The male doctor thought that gender-based violence, and many other sociocultural restrictions imposed in the name of religion, create many psychosocial problems for girls and women and even men and boys, and ultimately health is affected.

He believed that women and girls face nutritional deficiencies not because of poverty or resource constraints but largely due to the cultural notion that men and boys should eat more and be better fed.

He stated that medical doctors in any health care setting can only provide symptomatic treatment to a victim of violence; however, some passion-driven doctors can provide counselling services.

> "We tell the husband not to be violent."

Reported gender-based violence related experience

Being a senior doctor, the respondent believed that he, along with all other experienced doctors, has the capacity to identify hidden symptoms of gender-based violence and abuses such as physical, psychological and sexual abuse by husbands and in-laws. However, due to non-recognition of gender-based violence as a health issue, there is no official obligation and thus, in spite of being aware of the agony of the victim, as a doctor he cannot do much other than offering symptomatic treatment and referring the patient to a tertiary care hospital when deemed necessary.

He was of the view that doctors at present are not in a position to facilitate any legal aid or offer effective psychosocial counselling. Moreover, he thought that a male doctor is more limited in his role because women victims are monitored by male and female relatives, including the perpetrator (the husband) and it is not wise and socially acceptable to intervene in such matters.

Integration of services for gender-based violence

The respondent stated that domestic violence and other forms of violence such as rape cannot currently be addressed within a facility in "totality" because of "lack of knowledge and awareness of the doctors".

He added that there is no record-keeping on cases of gender-based violence in the health facility as there is no concept of it other than in medico-legal cases.

> "Unlike nongovernmental organizations who keep an exaggerated record of violence against women, we do not have any record."

In his view, the lady health worker who is so much respected that she is the *"baji"* (elder sister) in the community is the "bridge" between the victim/woman and the health system.

He stated that services such as counselling must be embedded in antenatal care facilities, to address issues of violence as pregnant women also suffer a lot. Battering of pregnant wives is usually on the grounds of "demand of a son".

In his opinion, gender-based violence can only be integrated in the health sector if there is information about it in the syllabus of medical education and training courses of lady health visitors, lady health workers and paramedics and overall, the country is in need of reforms in the education sector.

Gender-based violence, the health sector and the post-flood scenario

The male doctor was of the view that gender-based violence has increased during the floods and in the post-flood scenario because males are jobless and under severe stress and so the women, who are always the weaker ones, are the victims. He thought that gender-based violence had increased more among those flood affectees who had returned back to their homes because men find it easier to batter or torture their wives in the domestic setting than during their camp stay, where it was less likely. However, he did not exclude the possibility of incidents of violence against women and girls in the camps but said that these might have been kept "private".

He strongly believed that "our health sector" is capable of dealing with the needs of all the half million flood-affected pregnant women and can address the health needs of children of all ages, young and old. He cited the example of rural health centre A, where he was serving, and remarked how efficiently it is facing the challenge of increased turnover of patients in the outpatient department and in the antenatal clinic.

He argued that public sector facilities at the primary and secondary level of care are in fact "underutilized".

He was of the view that there are neither support mechanisms nor links with other line departments and voluntary organizations to address the issues of gender-based violence and that all facilities and line departments work independently and in isolation.

Gender-based violence and the medico-legal system

The respondent had learnt about certain laws to protect women through television advertisements but had never received any guidance from the health department in connection with gender-based violence.

Key findings from the lady health visitor's interview[27]

Gender-based violence and health-related considerations

The respondent said that the beating of wives in early marriages is very common in remote areas, where women are treated only as servants.

Like the preceding health service providers, she identified the very limited role of health service providers in addressing the complex problem of gender-based violence.

Reported gender-based violence related experience

The lady health visitor had seen cases of abuse due to domestic violence but was not able to offer any tangible help. She had referred some cases to medical doctors but she was not happy with the attitude of the doctors, especially that of the male doctors.

---

[27] Interviewed on 5 November 2010.

Integration of services for gender-based violence

The respondent said that currently there was no integration of services for gender-based violence but that such an integration, especially at antenatal clinics, may not only provide some help to the poor victims of violence, who are also very anaemic during pregnancy, but may also produce some well-trained health workers.

Gender-based violence, the health sector and the post-flood scenario

The respondent had no experience in the flood scenario but she commented that the health sector is not at all prepared to manage half a million pregnant women affected by floods. She identified the health needs of affectees of different age groups and pointed out that they also had needs that lie outside the health sector, such as shelter, clothing, cash and access to justice.

She was not aware of any support mechanisms and links.

Gender-based violence and the medico-legal system

The lady health visitor had some vague idea about laws to protect women and expected that the Government could take strong measures to change the situation and condition of women in remote areas of Sindh.

Key findings from the lady health worker's interview[28]

Gender-based violence and health-related considerations

"Hum bol nahin saktay." (We cannot speak for the victims of violence.)

The respondent had ample knowledge of different forms of violence against women and girls, was well aware of the local culture and articulated the same limitations that were shared by the other health service providers who were interviewed earlier.

Consequently, despite knowing the issues, she cannot go beyond first-aid treatment or counselling as a remedial gesture for the victims of domestic violence.

Reported gender-based violence related experience

Although cases of rape and assault exist in the community, they are not brought to the facility where she reports. However, she claimed that she can always recognize a case of domestic abuse, with or without physical injury, and these appear on a daily basis.

Integration of services for gender-based violence

The respondent confirmed the absence of record-keeping systems on gender-based violence.

Gender-based violence, health sector and the post-flood scenario

The respondent had no experience in the post-flood scenario but commented that the health sector is not at all prepared to manage half a million pregnant women affected by floods.

She was not aware of any support mechanisms and links.

---

[28] Interviewed on 5 November 2010.

Gender-based violence and the medico-legal system

She knew about medico-legal cases that were referred from her health centre to the Civil Hospital in Hyderabad.

Jamshoro district, Sindh

Key findings from the female doctor's interview [29]

Gender-based violence and health-related considerations

The respondent thought that medical doctors can only offer counselling services and symptomatic treatment to a woman victim of violence and that the violence is frequently caused by lack of education and unemployment.

She also stated that women of childbearing age suffer from anaemia and complications of pregnancy, and that young girls experience nutritional deficiencies due to culturally determined nutritional practices.

She thought that neglecting health care means that a woman's health deteriorates further and that when she suffers from violence from her husband the consequence is tragic and morally incorrect.

> "Because of domestic violence in which women are not only beaten but are not given money for everyday needs, complications take place – women turn into prostitutes under compulsion – sometimes their husbands even ask them to do so."

Reported gender-based violence related experience

The respondent has experience of working with women victims of violence, including minor girls, but in the latter case the mother or another relative tells the history. She finds it easy to refer complicated cases to the teaching hospital, which is within the campus of the dispensary where she is based.

She was of the view that a doctor cannot do much for a victim but "we can offer counselling – tell the woman to compromise".

Integration of services for gender-based violence

The female doctor was of the opinion that health facilities at all levels can address the problem of conjugal or domestic violence by addressing the physical ailments but not the actual causes of the violence as there is no such thing in the job descriptions of the health service providers; hence there is no record-keeping on gender-based violence. She thought that all health professionals can have a role in tackling the issues of gender-based violence, provided they are trained and possess the required skills.

She also thought that services for gender-based violence should include transport services and the entry point should be the antenatal clinics. In her view, the role of doctors is limited and lady health workers are in a better position to motivate an expectant mother to attend antenatal check-ups, or her mother-in-law to allow her to do so.

---

[29] Interviewed on 4 November 2010.

Gender-based violence, the health sector and the post-flood scenario

The respondent said that there had been incidents of sexual violence in the camps and that the women suffer nutritional deficiency as the food offered is only rice. She was of the opinion that the current state of the health sector was too weak to address the needs of half a million pregnant women who have been affected by the floods. She also thought that the health sector in Pakistan is incapable of fully addressing the health needs of different age groups, in both normal and disaster situations.

Gender-based violence and the medico-legal system

The respondent thought that the medico-legal system is the way to help the victims of violence.

Key findings from the male doctor's interview[30]

Gender-based violence and health-related considerations

The male doctor seldom deals with women patients and the victims of violence are usually women.

> "I recognize violence but I cannot offer help – how can I?"

The respondent claimed that male doctors have to be very careful when dealing with women patients socially.

He also thought that women do not give a correct history and usually only feel comfortable discussing gynaecological problems with female doctors. He stated that abortion is one factor that affects a woman's health and it is not much talked about, remaining hidden because of sociocultural communication barriers.

He thought that depression is a widely neglected consequence of gender-based violence.

Reported gender-based violence related experience

The respondent said that, although doctors have some experience in attending cases of violence, they can only offer symptomatic treatment. He thought that too much probing or interest by a doctor is not socially recommended and can cause anger and even suspicion among male members of the woman victim's family.

> "These days I notice elderly people who are malnourished – maybe this is also a violence?"

The respondent said that he finds no difficulty, socially or administratively, in referring medico-legal cases to the teaching hospital.

Integration of services for gender-based violence

The male doctor endorses the idea of integrating remedial services for gender-based violence at the antenatal clinic and believes that currently a health facility cannot address issues of domestic or conjugal violence because doctors can only offer symptomatic medical care.

---

[30] Interviewed on 4 November 2010.

Gender-based violence, the health sector and the post-flood scenario

The respondent was not attending any camp for flood affectees, so could not comment on questions related to the flood scenario. However, he thought that the health sector in Pakistan is capable of meeting the health needs of all kinds of patients and clients.

He said that no record-keeping for gender-based violence is practiced but that resources such as female staff, easy availability of mobile phones and field presence of lady health workers, are relevant and can be used to address issues of gender-based violence at the health facility level.

The respondent was of the view that multisectoral links are also potential resources, although at present they do not exist.

Gender-based violence and the medico-legal system

The respondent believed that the laws are in place but need to be implemented to protect women against violence.

Key findings from the lady health visitor's interview[31]

Gender-based violence and health-related considerations

> "Ham dartay hain." (We are scared.)

The respondent clearly pointed out that in a society and culture where women are abused on a daily basis in a variety of forms, and where male doctors are often rude with patients and support staff, how can one expect a lady health visitor to take the initiative and help a victim of violence other than giving first-aid treatment?

Reported gender-based violence related experience

> *"Wo hamary pas atay kab hain un ko ghar say bahar hee nahin nikala jata."* (The victims do not approach us – they are not allowed to leave their homes.)

The respondent disclosed her experience of attending cases of violence. She attended those cases with much secrecy and fear. However, she was of the view that if lady health visitors are given proper training, they are intelligent and committed enough to deal with such cases.

Integration of services for gender-based violence

The lady health visitor thought that there is no such integration at present and that pregnant women are neglected and abused, so it is a good idea to start extra services to help these women. She also thought that basic health units should be better equipped and that standards should be raised.

Gender-based violence, the health sector and the post-flood scenario

The respondent had no experience in the post-flood scenario and was unaware of any support mechanisms and links.

Gender-based violence and the medico-legal system

She had no knowledge of laws or policies to combat violence against women.

---

[31] Consent not given to include the name in the list of the respondents. Interviewed on 4 November 2010.

Key findings from the lady health worker's interview [32]

Gender-based violence and health-related considerations

The respondent was conscious of the barriers for lady health workers in addressing the issues of violence against women, which in her experience included *watta satta* (also known as *adla-badla* – an exchange marriage whereby a brother's sister is married to his wife's brother), honour killing and early marriage.

She thought that common beliefs and norms are against women and girls and that health measures such as contraception, which can reduce harm or bring improvement to a woman's life, are rejected in the name of Islamic injunctions.

> "I met a couple who have 11 children and when I talked to her and her husband about family planning, the husband refused."

> *"Jee bilkul jab hum family planning ki bat karnay gaon gothon mein jatay hain to especially molvi hazrat humain bohat bura bhala kahtay hain, 'tum log yahoodion ka kam kar rahay ho nikal jao humaray ghar say' tab ahsas hota hay kay jo female in kay sath rahti hain un kay sath kia hasher hoga."* (Yes, when we go from one village to another and pay home visits for creating awareness on family planning then men, especially male religious leaders of the mosque, criticize us severely and say "get out of our houses, you are implementing the agenda of Jews" and then we realize that those women who live with such men, what must they have been going through?)

The lady health worker said that women tend to seek health care from government hospitals but male doctors act quite rudely with female patients, especially girls, in the hospital's outpatient department. The women prefer traditional birth attendants, lady health visitors, lady health workers and quacks, who are easily accessible and are nice to them. However, she thought that boys and men have no problems and can visit any health care centre.

Reported gender-based violence related experience

The respondent narrated her experience of working with women and girl victims (minors, young and older women of childbearing age). She said that getting involved in violence-related issue of minor girls is problematic.

> *"Itna ziada nahin kyun ke un kay man bap kisi ko involve nahin karnay detaiy."* (Not so much – parents of the minor girls do not let others get involved.)

Being attached to a family planning programme, the respondent is usually with pregnant women who often suffer from missed abortions, life-threatening haemorrhages due to physical violence, and anaemia.

She said that she refers many pregnant women in labour or with physical injuries to the tertiary care hospital and has escaped any threat or pressure not to assist those women because "it always happened at night and I did not have to bother about legal issues".

---

[32] Consent not given to include the name in the list of the respondents. Interviewed on 3 November 2010.

She thought that lady health workers are the first level of contact for women victims of violence and that they can help the women to a great extent if they are dutiful and driven.

> *"Jee bilkul hum un ki help kartay hain un kay husband ya maan bap ko samjhatay hain aor un ki treatment bhi on the time hum log hi kartay hain bad mien wo jakay achay doctor ko dikhati hain."* (Yes we are the ones who help them (the women victims of violence), counsel their husbands or fathers and it is us who offer them timely first-aid treatment; later on they go to a good doctor.)

Integration of gender-based violence services

The respondent thought that integration of gender-based violence into the health sector to reduce violence is only possible when there are many rural health centres in all areas.

She said that women die during pregnancy as there is no transport to carry them to the tehsil headquarters or district headquarters hospitals. She also thought that women face a lot of violence, even during pregnancy, are overloaded with work and do not have the option to rest.

She thought that lady health workers currently do not maintain any records of incidents of gender-based violence, in spite of witnessing so much and doing a lot to address these issues, because of the understanding that "it is not our work".

Gender-based violence, the health sector and the post-flood scenario

The respondent was not aware of any incident of gender-based violence in camps and whether the government records had any option for recording gender-based violence in the camps.

She was of the view that the health sector cannot handle half a million flood-affected pregnant women and, similarly, is not capable of handling the needs of neonates, children, adolescents and young people. She pointed out that their needs include food, clothing, shelter, money and jobs, and that these are beyond the role of the health sector.

She was unaware of any support mechanisms and resources for health care providers/delivery staff to address cases of gender-based violence, including presence of female health care providers, self-safety mechanisms, skills and communication channels. Similarly, she was of the opinion that there are no existing health sector capacities or links with other sectors/line departments/civil society organizations to address issues of gender-based violence, including identifying gender-based violence, sensitive ways of communicating with patients, and responding to and documenting cases of gender-based violence.

Gender-based violence and the medico-legal system

The respondent had heard of some protection rights concerning women on television, but that was all. She did not think that the Government can take any effective action to control or reduce violence against women through the health sector.

Muzaffarabad district (Azad Jammu and Kashmir)

Key findings from the female doctor's interview[33]

Gender-based violence and health-related considerations

The female doctor was of the opinion that doctors face barriers and experience problems in the context of gender-based violence because there is "no policy to refer patients to police stations or any other relevant institutions".

She thought that the health care setting is extremely poor for all victims of violence (women/girls and boys/men), but especially for women and girls. She claimed that there is also a dire need to improve the relationship between patient and health staff.

Reported gender-based violence related experience

The respondent had experience of dealing with wife-battering cases and rape, including widows raped by in-laws. She lamented the problems involved in referral and reporting to police that discourage doctors to take an interest in helping victims of violence.

Integration of services for gender-based violence

The respondent was of the opinion that there is currently no integration of services but thought that antenatal clinics could be a good entry point as lady health visitors and lady health workers could provide counselling to the women.

She also said that the health sector has not yet developed a reporting system or referral mechanism for gender-based violence, as is the case with other departments, and that lack of awareness is prominent at the policy- and decision-making level. She thought that females are reluctant to share basic reasons for violence because of social pressures and also because the health facility does not offer any guarantee of privacy, confidentiality and practical help. She was also of the opinion that political parties are against ending gender-based violence and that higher authorities have no interest in this problem.

Gender-based violence, the health sector and the post-flood scenario

The respondent had observed that women even faced violence in camps and were overloaded with work, "fetching water for animals and for drinking while males are sleeping in their tents there".

She thought that owing to lack of "manpower" and other required resources, the health sector cannot meet the needs of either the half a million flood-affected pregnant women or of anybody else.

In her opinion, the health sector is devoid of support mechanisms and tangible resources.

Gender-based violence and the medico-legal system

She was unaware of any policy or law regarding gender-based violence. She thought that the

---

[33] Consent not given to include the name in the list of the respondents. Interviewed on 6 November 2010.

Government of Azad Jammu and Kashmir "must develop policies regarding gender-based violence and these should be implemented by the health department and other relevant authorities".

Key findings from the male doctor's interview[34]

Gender-based violence and health-related considerations

In the respondent's view, doctors and other health professionals are helpless and cannot do much about cases of rape, domestic violence and abuse, which are prevalent in Azad Jammu and Kashmir and caused by early marriage and the dowry systems.

The respondent's experience of dealing with women and girl victims in the health care setting includes cases presenting primarily with psychological issues due to violence. He added that boys and men present with physical pain due to corporal punishment by teachers or those in the workplace, while men also have mental and psychological issues due to the rapid change in socioeconomic conditions.

Reported gender-based violence related experience

> "Very rare cases surface, especially cases of sexual abuse, as they do not open the secret due to cultural barriers."

The male doctor thought that doctors can help, but are not allowed to due to social norms and absence of any protection to deal with cases of gender-based violence.

He also said that cases that fall under child protection are referred to the child protection complex for legal and psychological protection.

Integration of services for gender-based violence

The respondent thought that even though doctors do not have any policy guidelines or any incentives, the committed ones handle victims with great care within their available resources.

He thought that services, including counselling, medication, psychosocial support, self-protection and care, must be integrated at antenatal clinics to address the issues of violence and help victims.

Gender-based violence, the health sector and the post-flood scenario

The respondent concluded that women and girls face much psychosocial stress during floods, due to loss of family and property.

He believed that the district health departments and nongovernmental organizations jointly provide all the necessary basic facilities for pregnant women to eliminate their suffering, but "resources are very short and tragedy is great, and there is a need to do more".

Currently, there are no effective support mechanisms but "both Government, line departments and nongovernmental organizations should jointly establish a mechanism to be able to

---

[34] Consent not given to include the name in the list of the respondents. Interviewed on 6 November 2010.

establish well-equipped facilities, a database, registration processes, skilled manpower, women- and child-friendly spaces and psychosocial support activities – all these should be undertaken to address gender-based violence".

Gender-based violence and the medico-legal system

The respondent mentioned Azad Jammu and Kashmir's constitution and the Women and Children Rights Agency as instruments that are in place and can prevent violence against women.

> "Laws are very easy to constitute but very tough to implement, so implementation should be ensured by Government in all walks of life."

Key findings from the lady health visitor's interview[35]

Gender-based violence and health-related considerations

The respondent highlighted several forms of violence (e.g. local marriage customs in Azad Jammu and Kashmir), in addition to those given in the checklist. She favoured the role and involvement of lady health visitors in addressing the issues of violence against women, in spite of the known and unknown barriers, because she saw no other place for a woman who is suffering to go.

On a lighter note, she added that women do not choose to visit her health centre (rural health centre A) but rather insist to their husbands that they go to cities for the delivery of the baby as "it is their only excursion and why should they lose this opportunity"?

Reported gender-based violence related experience

The respondent has experience of dealing with women and girls who are in unhappy marriages and are mentally and physically tortured by their husbands and mother-in-laws.

> "I counsel them and tell them to remain patient and tolerant."

> "Unmarried women often used to come for abortions but now there are a lesser number of such women, as knowledge about contraception is common."

Integration of services for gender-based violence

The respondent was in complete agreement that the integration of services such as counselling and awareness about women's rights would benefit women.

She noted that, other than cases reported to police under "medico-legal", there is no record-keeping on violence against women.

She believed that the prevalence of gender-based violence would be reduced if the problem is addressed at health facilities, as the treatment, counselling and knowledge of their rights would give a voice and power to the helpless victims of violence.

---

[35] Interviewed on 8 November 2010.

Gender-based violence, the health sector and the post-flood scenario

> "I do not know of any link or coordination of the health sector with any other nongovernmental organization or department."

She articulated that the recent floods caused a decrease in "domestic violence" because all affectees were homeless and "men did not have any private space to beat up their wives in the open or even in the camp".

In spite of believing in the capacity of the health sector to deal with flood-affected pregnant women and neonates, she pointed out the absence of attention to the health needs of adolescents and young people within health care practice.

Gender-based violence and the medico-legal system

The respondent stated that she was unaware of any specific laws to protect women or guidelines to treat victims of violence.

Key findings from the lady health worker's interview[36]

> "Kashmiri women are suffering badly from violence at every stage of life."

Gender-based violence and health-related considerations

The respondent mentioned that in the villages, females are not allowed to marry the person whom they love and any woman who tries to exercise her free will faces both physical and psychological violence.

In addition, she said that the community does not allow girls to attend health awareness workshops and this creates a barrier for lady health workers in addressing issues of violence.

She pointed out that lack of awareness about body changes at different phases of their life imposes a health threat to women and girls. Also, boys are hesitant to attend health facilities to discuss sexual health problems, while men are arrogant and lack correct knowledge of religion. She believed that these factors impact on the health of a woman in her different roles and at different phases of her life.

Reported gender-based violence related experience

The respondent did not disclose her experience of dealing with cases of violence against women. However, there was a suggestion that she had witnessed such cases.

She said that there is no advantage in bringing up issues of violence at a health facility because "her relatives will become our enemy".

Integration of services for violence against women

The respondent said that she cannot imagine any such services because neither a woman doctor nor any antenatal clinic exists in her geographic area.

---

[36] Consent not given to include the name in the list of the respondents. Interviewed on 8 November 2010.

Gender-based violence, the health sector and the post-flood scenario

The respondent had some experience of working with flood-affected women and violence is nothing new to them. She was disappointed with the capacity of the health sector to address the needs of a large number of patients from different age groups.

Gender-based violence and the medico-legal system

She had witnessed one medico-legal case but the police were helpless before the angry father and brother who were the perpetrators of the violence.

She had not heard of any law or policy in connection with violence against women.

Kasur district, Punjab

Key findings from the female doctor's interview[37]

In this interview, most of the responses regarding gender-based violence were in sharp contrast with those shared by the other health service providers.

Gender-based violence and health-related considerations

> "Violence against women? Women are no longer simple and stupid. I see criminal women who have killed their husbands, have multiple partners and there are girls who, after being dumped in an otherwise consensual relationship, present themselves as a victim. I see alleged and fabricated rape cases."

However, the female doctor acknowledged that some women do face violence, for instance there is a very strong desire for a son, therefore sex-selective abortion and "back street abortion" is very common.

She felt that doctors can address the issues of gender-based violence but if they do so they will face threats and their personal safety will be compromised.

She also said that dealing with gender-based violence is not in the job description of doctors.

Reported gender-based violence related experience

Since the respondent bears the additional responsibility of being a medico-legal officer, she is "over loaded" with criminal cases and "is so stressed that I want to quit".

Integration of services for gender-based violence

The respondent was not convinced that violence against women is too prevalent.[38] She identified poor finances and greed as the causes of specific forms of violence whereby men use women for commercial sex purposes or drug trafficking.

> "Women get concessions in the law, therefore they are used by men for their crimes."

---

[37] Consent not given to include the name in the list of the respondents. Interviewed on 10 November 2010.
[38] Kasur is among one of the 15 districts of Pakistan with the most reported cases of violence against women (Perveen, 2010).

Gender-based violence and the medico-legal system

The respondent was well aware of the medico-legal system but her stance on gender-based violence is very strong and clear. She pointed out that distractions from Islam also create such problems in society.

Key findings from the male doctor's interview [39]

Gender-based violence and health-related considerations

> "Property disputes and preferences for a son are the sociocultural factors that also contribute to harming the health of women in our environment."

The respondent thought that gender-based violence is a very private matter and doctors do not wish to be party to it.

In his opinion, women suffer from various forms of violence and do not have many choices. He thought that even today, the practice of nutritional discrimination is strong in our society.

He pointed out interesting dichotomies in the conduct of woman. According to his observation and experience, women who usually face mobility restriction somehow find it relatively easy to visit or seek permission to visit a health facility. Younger women prefer to see male doctors and women of all ages usually trust a male physician more than a female doctor.

> "They need an emotional catharsis."[40]

Reported gender-based violence related experience

The respondent had experience of dealing with cases of gender-based violence. He had even dealt with a rape of a four-year-old girl who required extensive surgical procedures.

> "Such cases reveal the torn moral fabric of our society."

Integration of services for gender-based violence

He endorses the idea of integrating services to cater for issues of gender-based violence, especially at the antenatal clinics, but is not in favour of creating vacancies for counsellors.

Gender-based violence and the capacity of the health sector

In his opinion, the health sector has no capacity to address the health needs of all those who are in need.

Gender-based violence and the medico-legal system

The male doctor thought nothing can be specified, although there is a lot of noise in the media. The Government should be "strict on legal proceedings and have a proper monitoring system".

---

[39] Interviewed on 10 November 2010.
[40] This view is interesting, as it counters the conventional view that women prefer to see female doctors. However, in our assessment of Kasur in 2006, the women in the communities expressed the same ... that they had no particular preference whether they saw female or male doctors. It was the men of the community who indicated that they wanted their women to only see female doctors.

Key findings from the lady health visitor's interview[41]

Gender-based violence and health-related considerations

> *"Bhai kehtay hain tum nay hissa kiyun manga jo mangay uss say rishta khatam yeh bhi zulm hay."* (Brothers question their sister on how she dare ask for her inheritance right and those who insist and finally take it up experience a social boycott – this is also violence.)

The respondent recognized, but could not address, gender-based violence at the health facility level.

> "Who knows why there was a 'stove burst' and she was abused – was it because she brought a lesser than expected dowry? What can be done by a lady health visitor?"

Reported gender-based violence related experience

As a practicing lady health visitor and trainer, she had experience of seeing and dealing with cases of stove burns, acid burns, suicide, drowning and homicides.

Integration of services for gender-based violence

The respondent emphasized that the training needs of lady health visitors and lady health workers must be assessed: they should be trained so that they can contribute towards addressing remedies for gender-based violence within health care settings.

Gender-based violence and the capacity of the health sector

The respondent was of the view that, in addition to increasing the capacity of the health sector through training of different levels of health service providers, opinion shapers such as the imams of mosques must be involved for an overall change in the societal attitude towards the issue of gender-based violence.

Gender-based violence and the medico-legal system

Like most of the preceding respondents, the respondent had heard "something" on television but could not specify any law or policy to address violence against women. She emphasized the Government's role in this issue and urged the inclusion of other players to examine the problem of violence against women and girls in Kasur and across the country.

Key findings from the lady health worker's interview[42]

Gender-based violence and health-related considerations

The respondent thought that if lady health workers offer "too much" assistance to the victim of violence, they may face social pressures, especially from the victim's family.

She thought that people are unaware of the issue and also do not cooperate.

---

[41] Interviewed on 10 November 2010.
[42] Interviewed on 10 November 2010.

In her opinion, women can seek family planning services far more easily than men and that women seek health care from soothsayers and traditional healers (*pirs* and *faquirs*) in the first instance, rather than from trained health care providers.

She said that boys and young men are encouraged to see a doctor because the family feels that they need proper treatment as "they are the earning hands of a family".

Reported gender-based violence related experience

The respondent reported that she has been helping young married women who face verbal and physical abuse, for example from a dowry being less than expected or from the demands for a son, and counsels them and their mothers directly.

> "Recently I advised a newly wed not to accept the threat of divorce from her lawyer husband and his pressure to her parents to give him more money. She and her mother listened to me. Her husband left her at her parent's home and when, contrary to his calculation, he did not find any outcome of his threat, he finally decided to take her back."

However, she accepted that not all these stories have happy endings and that lady health workers can be at risk if they take too much interest in a case.

Integration of services for gender-based violence

> "What is the use of giving awareness to women; how can women tell men not to beat them? Men need to be trained and become aware of issues of violence. Had they been wise, why should they have become abusers?"

The respondent liked the idea of integration but articulated her fear that if husbands who are abusers come to know that doctors at the health facility are keen to address the issues of violence, they may fear police or legal action against them and will stop their wives visiting any health facility.[43]

> "*Rahi sahi aazadi bhi khatam.*" (Whatever freedom women have would also be ended then.)

She said that currently there is no practice, or even thought, of recognizing and registering a cases of violence against women at the health facility level and no mention of dealing with gender-based violence in a lady health worker's job description.

In her opinion, antenatal clinics are good and safe points for integrating services for addressing gender-based violence as "there are all women around".

Besides health service providers, she thought the imams of mosques should be involved in educating men.

Gender-based violence and capacity of the health sector

The respondent thought that the public health sector does not have enough capacity to liaison with other line departments and civil society organizations.

---

[43] A very important point to keep in mind and this must be discussed with stakeholders and the duty bearers.

Gender-based violence and the medico-legal system

The respondent said that she was aware of the law for harassment against women at the workplace through television.

The questions related to floods were irrelevant for Kasur-based respondents as Kasur district did not flood and therefore there were no camps for internally displaced persons. However, some respondents were aware of the increase in incidence of gender-based violence during floods and in camp settings. Sexual torture and rape was specifically mentioned in the Bhakkar, Layyah, Muzaffargarh and Mianwali districts of Punjab.

Table 1. Quantification of 20 queries for the 20 health service providers from four districts with a brief qualitative analysis.

No.	Query	Yes	No	Any other response/comments
1.	Do you think you would face any barriers in addressing gender-based violence/violence against women as a health service provider?	15	05	Even those who said "Yes" identified the limited role that they could actually offer
2.	Would you like to identify key sociocultural factors that influence health of women/girls and men/boys in your area of work?	20	00	Women and girls were more influenced and affected by such factors
3.	Can women access and use health facilities and services as easily as men?	15	05	Both men and women could access these facilities with equal ease or difficulty, according to the situation
4.	Would you like to identify certain health and social outcomes and consequences of negligence of health considerations for women/girls and boys/men?	20	00	None of the respondents could think of any problem for men and boys
5.	Have you ever worked with clients/patients who may have been victims of violence?	20	00	Other than lady health visitors and lady health workers, health service providers did not recognize cases of violence as gender-based violence/violence against women
6.	Do you think health service providers who suspect that a patient is a victim of conjugal or sexual violence would usually ask their patient about it?	00	20	Health service providers may have suspected but they rarely asked questions or intervened. Their degree of interest and ability to look into these issues decreased with increasing seniority and level of the health service provider
7.	Do you believe you could help a woman who is a victim of violence?	13	07	Helping was mostly equated to medical treatment and counselling was equated to an emphasis on compromise with the violence, or on ignoring the crime due to social norms
8.	Do you refer cases of violence?	20	00	Health service providers maintained that they

No.	Query	Yes	No	Any other response/comments
9.	Do you think that a client who uses antenatal care services might be at risk for any of the types of violence mentioned before?	12	08	always referred cases where necessary Antenatal clinics were thought to be the best entry point for integrating such services, as married women face a lot of domestic violence
10.	Is the record-keeping system equipped to register and monitor incidents of gender-based violence?	00	20	There is no such thing in the job description of any health service provider and there is no such requirement in the reporting mechanisms. Thus, in practice this becomes an invalid query[44]
11.	Are there any support mechanisms and existing resources for health care providers/delivery staff to address cases of gender-based violence, including presence of female health care providers, self-safety mechanisms, skills, communication channels?	05	15	Support mechanisms were not clear to health service providers. Even the existence of female workers, access to mobile phones or knowledge of self-safety mechanisms were not considered support mechanisms or resources in the context of addressing gender-based violence/violence against women and girls
12.	Are there any existing health sector capacities and links with other sectors/line departments/civil society organizations to address gender-based violence, including identifying gender-based violence, sensitive ways of communicating with patients on gender-based violence (e.g. capacity to engage victims in conversation), responding to and documenting cases of gender-based violence?	17	03	Those who said "Yes" also emphasized the weakness of such links
13.	Did you notice any incidence of gender-based violence/violence against women and girls during and after floods?	10	10	There were mixed views, as not all health service providers were involved in flood relief activities
14.	Do you think the health sector is prepared to manage half a million pregnant women who are affected by floods?	15	05	Those who said "Yes" thought it was in fact also a measure of their own performance

---

[44] This will be a challenge to address and operationalize in the standard operating procedures but extremely important to push forward on documentation. Perhaps lady health workers can begin the process but only with strong support, protection and with confidentiality ensured.

No.	Query	Yes	No	Any other response/comments
15.	Do you think the health sector is prepared to address the needs (kindly specify the needs as well) of flood-affected neonates, infants and children?	15	05	There was no clear and common understanding among health service providers about the age of children. There was no attention to the specific needs of male and female children. Transgenders were virtually excluded
16.	Do you think the health sector is prepared to address the needs of flood-affected adolescents and youth?	20	00	There was no clear understanding of the issues of adolescents and young people. There was no attention to the specific needs of males and females. Transgenders were virtually excluded
17.	Are you aware of national policies or laws that exist to prevent violence against women?	15	05	Those who said "Yes" could not specify or explain any law or policy. Those who said "Yes" had heard of some women protection bills and laws, especially on harassment, through television but nobody was clear or very knowledgeable
18.	Are you aware of laws or policies that require specific actions by health service providers with regard to violence against women?	00	20	All health service providers, however, were familiar with medico-legal terms and the problems involved due to the attitude of the police, community, family members and, ultimately, court hearings
19.	Do you think it is the role of the Government to address the problem of violence against women?	15	05	Health service providers suggested training and monetary incentives as remedial measures for improving the performance of the providers besides urging multisectoral, especially the education sector's, involvement in these issues
20.	Do you see any challenges in integrating gender-based violence in the health sector?	17	03	Resistance from the community was the commonest challenge identified

Reflections from the discussion with the participants of a two-day WHO training workshop in August 2010

Participants of the three group discussions[45] were selected from health service providers who attended a two-day training workshop on gender conducted by WHO Pakistan in August 2010 in four districts (Jamshoro and Dadu, Sindh; Muzaffarabad, Azad Jammu and Kashmir; and Kasur, Punjab) where the Basic Development Needs Programme is working.

The main objective of this exercise was to gain an insight into the perceptions and perspectives of these relatively well-trained health service providers without evaluating the accuracy of their

---

[45] Discussions were held on 4 November 2010 in Jamshoro, Sindh; 8 November 2010 in Muzaffarabad, Azad Jammu and Kashmir; and 10 November 2010 in Kasur, Punjab.

knowledge about gender, the gender–health nexus and gender-based violence, and without judging the quality of the training that materialized in a very short time on complex issues.

All sessions began with questions designed to create a rapport with the discussants. They were asked to share their reflections on the training they had received and how they felt about gender and gender-based violence in their areas of work.

The ice-breaking session was followed by a round of questions by the researcher and the discussants engaged in an interactive dialogue. The average discussion time for all discussions was 55–60 minutes.

The following account illustrates highlights of the discussion under the themes specified in the data collection instruments for this group (see methodology in Chapter 1 and Annex 1).

Links between gender-based violence and health at the policy level

Policies are not clear; therefore very few health service providers are aware of gender-based violence and related issues.

Only district headquarter and tehsil headquarter hospitals currently deal with cases of violence.

The effectiveness of links between gender-based violence and health at the policy level

Since knowledge and awareness of gender-based violence is almost negligible among health service providers, the effectiveness of any such links is non-existent or is not applicable to the current state of the health sector.

Links between gender-based violence and health at the legislation level

There is almost no awareness of laws and health legislation, even among senior members of the health sector. Overall, the guilty are rarely brought to justice and this contributes towards perpetuation of these crimes against women and girls.

The recent laws and legislation that have been put in place in Pakistan, such as the law on harassment against women or the bill on women's protection, do not exist in Azad Jammu and Kashmir.

The effectiveness of links between gender-based violence and health at the legislation level

Obviously, there is no question of any effective implementation of the laws if there is no law; if there is a law, nobody knows how to use it in favour of the victim of violence, who is usually a woman from a poor background in a socially disadvantaged position.

Links between gender-based violence and health at the operational level

The issues of gender-based violence should be integrated across the board in the health sector. Senior health officials, health workers and community members must be involved together to address this complex issue as society, culture, religion and economy all determine the patterns, prevalence and patronization of different expressions and manifestations of gender-based violence.

The effectiveness of links between gender-based violence and health at the operational level

No project or programme can be effective if there is no ownership from the community.

Links between gender-based violence and health at the guidelines level

No guidelines are available at any level of health service provision and hence there is almost a blindness, or silence, on issues of gender-based violence.

The effectiveness of links between gender-based violence and health at the guidelines level

Again, since there are no guidelines, the question of measuring their effectiveness is invalid.

In nearly all discussions, participants openly examined beliefs, attitudes, norms and value systems prevalent in the communities where they work. They appeared to confirm through their responses that they are in favour of women's rights, equality of gender and understand the role of the health sector and health service providers in addressing the issues of gender-based violence. However, they voiced certain risks, speculations and concerns about the point of view of those health service providers who are not sensitized, are unaware of the concept of gender and are opinion-makers in the communities.

Summary of "unsaid" questions raised by participants

- Why is the health sector suddenly interested in gender-based violence?
- If gender-based violence is a public health issue, why was it not conveyed to the health service providers much earlier?
- What are the incentives for the health service providers who take a risk and address gender-based violence?
- How will the media and nongovernmental organizations be kept within limits so that they do not exploit a victim for their own benefit and publicity?
- The community needs to be trained for changing their mindsets – is the health sector ready to allocate resources for interacting with the opinion-makers in the community and genuinely be involved at the grass-roots level?

Reflections from consultations (e-mail, telephone, face-to-face) with 10 public health experts within and outside WHO Pakistan

The opinions of the experts can broadly be divided into two groups: the proponents and opponents.

The proponents (six in number) endorse the idea of integration of gender-based violence into the health sector but they advise remaining cognizant of inherent deficiencies of the health sector and a very deficient intersectoral and multisectoral coordination.

All experts, including those who admired the infrastructure of the basic health units and rural health centres in Pakistan, are unsatisfied with:

- the levels of privacy in health centres;
- the way medical records are stored;
- the existing capacity of health service providers to maintain privacy and confidentiality;
- the administration and effectiveness of the referral systems;
- the capacity of the sector for medico-legal information;
- the capacity and resources available for consistent recording of cases of gender-based violence.[46]

However, the proponents point out that whatever appears as weaknesses can be translated into strengths (staff, infrastructure, etc.).

Others are sceptic about the reality of gender-based violence as a public health issue. In their view it is a social issue, outside the area of health.

Some selected responses

> "Frankly speaking, I have no experience of dealing with such cases in my professional life, but they do happen. I haven't come across them in hospital but I do hear about them from time to time, mostly on the media. Usually these patients have head injury or orthopaedic injuries or burns, in PIMS[47] not having these specialities I do not have a chance to see these patients. However, I would like to help further and, as I already said, this will educate me." (Senior specialist surgeon, PIMS, Islamabad, Pakistan)

> "In my opinion this (gender-based violence) issue has never been part of the health sector. Usually, issues of violence are seen as crimes and the health sector is not formatted to see this as its own indigenous problem." (Former female medical doctor, currently a civil servant, Sindh, Pakistan)

Structured observations by the researcher

Health sector structural readiness to address gender-based violence can be observed through:

- attitudes;

---

[46] A randomized survey among 100 obstetricians–gynaecologists in Pakistan in 2002 found that "the significant mismatch between perceptions of prevalence of domestic violence in Pakistani society (> 30%) and in clinical practice (< 10%) suggests that obstetricians are socially aware of the enormous public health burden but cannot associate an equivalent magnitude among their clientele". *Addressing violence against women* (http://www.whatworksforwomen.org/chapters/21/sections/59, accessed November 2010).
[47] Pakistan Institute of Medical Sciences (Islamabad-based tertiary care and teaching hospital).

- sensitivity;
- health service providers' fear of helping survivors of gender-based violence at health facilities and fear of addressing this issue as a "health problem".

Attitudes vary with different health service providers; however, men generally have a patriarchal mindset. Many woman health service providers also endorse subjugation of women, as may be validated by the counselling advice. The effect of negative perceptions of women, as evidenced in the literature, is always endorsed by sociocultural factors, in particular anti-woman and rape-supportive attitudes.

As in other developing countries, health service providers fear going beyond a certain limit. If health service providers take an interest in cases of domestic violence at all, they fear going beyond a certain limit as the violence happens in the sacred sphere of the family.

Levels of privacy

Levels of privacy in health centres include:

- effective sound and visual barriers;
- how medical records are stored and who has access to them;
- referrals (and awareness of) to available resources/support (medical, medico-legal, information).

There are no sound-proof rooms but there are separate rooms for female and male doctors and an examination area is separately allocated. However, in general, doctors do not care for the privacy of patients. The door remains open and other staff or visitors can intervene while the doctor is attending the patient. This practice, though not recommended even for routine examinations, is completely unacceptable when dealing with suspected or confirmed cases of gender-based violence.

Medical records are kept in designated registers and are placed on the doctor's table. Theoretically, these are only accessible to the doctor in charge but, in practice, the confidentiality of the records is seldom ascertained. Medico-legal certificates and documents are not even kept in a locked cabinet or drawer and any unauthorized staff can access them and misuse the information.

All health service providers are aware of the referral systems and procedures but, in practice, the referral system is not strong. In medico-legal cases, the concerned doctor cannot refer a case without going through the formalities of the procedure which, in turn, is only initiated when there is a letter from the police. Otherwise, cases of assault and injury remain unrecorded, if not unnoticed, as crimes of gender-based violence.

Capacity and resources available for consistent recording of cases of gender-based violence

Since there is no clause for recording gender-based violence, health service providers do not record it. Record registers or reporting at any level, or in any chain of command, do not require this specific record-keeping. Thus, health service providers, despite knowing through community contacts, examination or history that they are actually dealing with a case of gender-based violence, can never record it as such. Only those cases of violence that qualify as medico-legal are recorded and in many of these cases fabrication is practiced, either wilfully or under compulsion.

Chapter 4. Views and voices of women and men from the community from the four districts

This chapter presents the rapid assessment's findings regarding the health sector's readiness to integrate gender-based violence in Pakistan, including Azad Jammu and Kashmir, based on data collected from focus group discussions in the selected four districts with men and women (see methodology in Chapter 1).

The chapter is divided into three parts. The first part sums up the key findings in the light of the responses from the focus group discussions with the four groups of men, one from each of the four districts. The second part sums up key findings in the light of the responses from the focus group discussions with the four groups of women, one from each of the four districts. The third part assembles the overall impressions of the researcher, based on the groups' responses and her own observations. Tables 3 and 4 contain district-wise qualitative analysis of the focus group discussion with men and women from the community and give a quick review and understanding of the entire situation regarding gender-based violence and its integration into the health sector of Pakistan and Azad Jammu and Kashmir.

Findings from the focus group discussions with the men from the community[48]

Hyderabad district, Sindh

When asked the question "If a woman is living in a violent relationship or has experienced violence, how might she get help?" the general response was that "it is not possible to get help in our society".[49]

Use of any health facility and treatment options

General responses

The respondents frequently use public sector health facilities (dispensaries or hospitals) because fees are high in private clinics.

They usually use bus or rickshaw to take their children or other family members to a government hospital.

Usually, trained doctors are sought, as quacks, hakims and homeopaths are thought to be unreliable.

Two respondents mentioned motorbikes as the means of transport for carrying a patient to any health facility.

---

[48] Held on 3 November 2010 in Jamshoro, Sindh; 5 November 2010 in Hyderabad, Sindh; 6 November 2010 in Muzaffarabad, Azad Jammu and Kashmir; and 10 November 2010 in Kasur, Punjab.

[49] This implies that it is impossible for a woman to get out of an abusive relationship; marriage is a sacred institution and divorce is still a stigma.

Specific responses

One respondent said that a private health facility is preferred as they are not satisfied with government-sector health facilities.

Health care for pregnant women

General responses

Men support women in accessing health care during pregnancy.

Men support women in accessing family planning services.

Specific responses:

> "But some Pathan families don't support their women to access health facilities during pregnancies."

> "No, most people did not observe family planning in the past but nowadays, because of the poverty, people are doing this."

Violence – general views

General responses

The terminology "gender-based violence/violence against women" was not recognized in Urdu or English.

Following an explanation of the concepts, the respondents were of the opinion that these cases and practices of violence against women and girls happen in "most places" but they are "heard less" as they are concealed and the community feels it is a very private matter and disclosure is equal to loss of honour.

Often, married women are beaten by in-laws collectively because of property disputes after the woman's father dies.

The respondents also pointed out a geographical distribution of the violence and emphasized an urban/rural division.

Owing to access to mass media they are aware of those cases of violence against women and girls that had been highlighted in the media, especially on private television channels.

Specific responses

> "There is a person – my neighbour – he once beat his wife very badly and when we tried to stop him, he also tried to fight with me and said it was their 'home matter'; he used to beat her because he drinks alcohol daily and his income is less and whenever his wife asks for money or something for the kids, he starts to beat her."

> "Violence is a common experience in the lives of women in our district and city but it is less in cities and more in the rural and remote areas."

> "We hear and read daily that this is happening in Pakistan, just like *karo kari* (honour killing) or divorce, because of dowry and girls are bearing violence from their in-laws."

> "Girls cannot walk alone at night (after 8 p.m.)."

Gender-based violence and health facilities

General responses

All respondents have experience of taking "someone" to a health facility but only a few respondents voluntarily disclosed that they had ever taken a victim of violence from their families to any health facility and those were males[50] who were the victims and had been badly beaten by their in-laws. They took the victims to a private hospital where medicines and minor surgical treatment were offered and they were satisfied with the treatment.

However, there is a consensus that more women are beaten and maltreated by their in-laws and husbands and they do not like this conduct and practice.

Specific responses

> "One day we were in the civil hospital in Hyderabad and we saw a female who was badly hurt by the husband but the hospital management were not treating her, they were saying that 'it is a police case and we cannot do any thing unless the police come'. The girl was crying with pain."

> "It is not a good experience and we have to avoid this type of activity because before doing this we must think also that we have sisters and daughters."

Jamshoro district, Sindh

> "*Bevas uthan bar chadya*" – a Sindhi proverb quoted by a participant to reflect on the situation of women and health facilities. (When things go beyond one capacity, even mighty animals surrender to the situation.)

Use of any health facility and treatment options

General responses

Respondents visit health care facilities often due to illness and accidents. They generally use local transport and occasionally a taxi or rickshaw. The preference for a delivery case is either a *dai* or traditional birth attendant or a gynaecologist in a private clinic.

Health care for pregnant women

General responses

Men support women in accessing health care during pregnancy.

Men support women in accessing family planning services.

---

[50] In violent subcultures this happens too. However, the frequency, or at least the reported one, is less than the reported cases of violence against women. Further, such conversations and even the media reports seldom, if ever, disclose the contextual details or reasons leading to beating or manhandling of male members.

Specific responses

> "Due to my wife's delivery I visited a government facility, and that was my last experience because it was a bad experience, because the female doctor came after four hours."

Violence – general views and gender-based violence and health facilities

General responses

The terminology "gender-based violence/violence against women" was not recognized in Sindhi, Urdu or English. Following an explanation of the concepts, the respondents were of the opinion that these incidents did not happen in reality.

On probing, the respondents came up with marriage customs like early marriages, *watta satta*, property disputes, honour killing, and need and desire for an heir (*waris*) as the causes of violence against women and girls.

Specific responses

> "Yes, but now it is less."

> "I have seen it in early marriages."

> "*Choti choti baton par bewiyon par tashadud.*" (Battering of wives for trivia.)

> "*Bachiyon ko school na bhejna bhi zulm hay.*" (Depriving girls of schooling is also a violence.)

If a woman is living in a violent relationship or has experienced violence, how might she get help?

General responses

The general opinion was that a woman should compromise and accept the situation.

Specific responses

> "*Uss nay sabar karna hota hay aor zindagi bachon ki waja say guzarni hoti hay.*" (The woman has to exercise patience and lead her life with compromises because of the kids.)

Gender-based violence and health facilities

The men did not open up and nothing more relevant than what was shared earlier could be retrieved.

A general response was "yes, we do consult the health care centres but only rarely because this violence has to be and is resolved in jirga".

They also hinted at the powerless position of the health service providers.

"They – all health providers – are in fear from both parties."

Muzaffarabad district, Azad Jammu and Kashmir

Use of any health facility and treatment options and health care for pregnant women

Their responses are almost the same as those of the men from Hyderabad and Jamshoro. However, the respondents prefer to be treated by a trained medical doctor at the health facility and are not happy with the overall attitude of the doctors and paramedics towards the patients. They share the view that men, including themselves, are caring husbands and offer all possible support to women when they are unwell, especially during pregnancy.

Violence – general views and gender-based violence and health facilities

The respondents did not open up much. They were of the view that in their city there cannot be more than 30% cases of violence and that the media gives an exaggerated picture. An interesting but alarming (though in conformity with the patriarchal mindset) justification for violence against women and girls was that those women who do not "obey men" become the victims of violence.

Following an explanation of the concepts of gender-based violence/violence against women and girls by the researcher/moderator, some respondents emphasized the role of the deteriorating economy in causing different forms of violence.

Since the men were in denial and not ready to open up, no information could be retrieved on any experience of cases of violence at the level of the health facility. However, two respondents mentioned corporal punishment given to children at school.

Some respondents talked in detail about the issues of child labour and wondered why it was being sidelined while violence against women and girls was being given so much attention.

Kasur district, Punjab

Use of any health facility and treatment options

General responses

The community frequently uses the district headquarter and tehsil headquarter hospitals and usually uses motorcycles, rickshaws or local vans to get there, as the approximate distance to the nearest public health facility is 8 km.

Specific responses

"We often visit public health sector facilities due to the low cost of treatment."

"Due to the short distance of the public health facility from our residence."

"The community can't afford costly treatment in the private hospital."

"I prefer the traditional healers due to low cost of treatment."

> "Poor people cannot afford the private facility."

Health care for pregnant women

General responses

Mostly, articulated responses were similar to those in Sindh and Azad Jammu and Kashmir regarding the support and care of pregnant wives.

Specific responses

> "We can't support a proper check-up like an ultrasound check-up because there is no facility in tehsil headquarters and basic health units."

> "We can support more if we are properly aware about the family planning facility."

Violence – general views

General responses

As elsewhere, the respondents were unaware of the terms and concepts "gender-based violence/violence against women". However, following an explanation by the moderator, most of the participants said that these types of violence often happen in their villages.

Violence is common in women's lives, due to the financial crisis (said by two participants), and drug addiction of husbands and low educational background were considered the reasons behind beating wives with a "stick". Another form of violence mentioned was "acid throwing".

Specific response

> "It (i.e. beating or verbal abuse) only happens after frequent births of daughters."

Gender-based violence and health facilities

The respondents had no experience of taking any woman or male victim of violence to a health facility.

However, they stressed urgent improvement of the quality and availability of services and free medicines so that the poor can benefit.

All respondents had a consensus that medical officers, nurses and lady health visitors could be helpful and respond to cases of violence if they wanted to.

Findings from the focus group discussions with the women from the community[51]

Hyderabad district, Sindh

> "Why did God make me a female, it is really painful?" (A respondent in the focus group discussions)

Use of any health facility and treatment options

The women's responses were almost the same as those of the men from Hyderabad. This reflects that men and women at least communicate on certain matters besides underscoring male dependency on the mobility decisions of women.

General responses

The respondents frequently use public sector health facilities (dispensaries or hospitals) because fees are high in private clinics.

The respondents usually use wagons, buses or rickshaws to take their children or other family members to a government hospital. Trained doctors are usually sought out, as quacks, hakims and homeopaths are not reliable.

Two respondents mentioned motorbikes and cars as the means of transport for carrying a patient to a health facility.

Private health facilities are preferred as the educated respondents are not satisfied with government sector health facilities.

Specific responses

> "Unemployment in Pakistan is the major reason that the people go to government health facilities and in private clinics, fees are higher and we can't afford them. We are always unsatisfied with these government facilities."

> "Sometimes we have to consult any non-doctor to save time and money but they are not reliable."

Health care for pregnant women

General responses

Men support women in accessing health care during pregnancy but sometimes they do not because "it all depends on their mood".

Men support women in accessing family planning services in these times of high inflation.

---

[51] Held on 3 November 2010 in Jamshoro, Sindh; 5 November 2010 in Hyderabad, Sindh; 6 November 2010 in Muzaffarabad, Azad Jammu and Kashmir; and 10 November 2010 in Kasur, Punjab.

Violence – general views

General responses

The terminology "gender-based violence/violence against women" was not recognized in Urdu or English. Three women in the discussion group started weeping when the moderator explained gender-based violence. One of them said "we are in the list of all forms of violence".

Following an explanation of the concepts, the respondents were of the opinion that a female is "made for violence".

The most common forms of violence for the respondents are sexual violence, sexual abuse and domestic violence.

It is a common experience but not commonly disclosed.

Like men, women are also aware of many stories of rape and abduction, currently highlighted on television channels.

Responding to the query, "If a woman is living in a violent relationship or has experienced violence, how might she get help?" the consensus was that, because of societal norms, nothing can be done to help her.

Specific responses

"In childhood she faces brother and father domination, and after marriage this right or duty is taken over by her husband and in-laws."

"Domestic violence is always borne by females but after marriage we face many other types of violence, like sexual or physical abuse."

"Males always want to put down females, and there is always an ego problem in every matter when females say something."

"It is much more here as well because I am suffering from these things and other females in my neighbourhood or family discuss this with me but they cannot do anything to help me practically."

"It happens with me daily – my husband sexually uses me in a bad way (anal sex) which is not allowed in Islam but I cannot do anything because when I say something he starts beating me."

"I tried (to escape to get a divorce) but in Pakistan no one supported me – they said that I had a child, etc."

Gender-based violence and health facilities

General responses

All have experienced violence. The opinion was that "this is one thing which we pray not to experience".

According to three respondents, being in a hospital or any other government facility is seldom a good experience and most of the time it is bad because "the lower management do not know how to talk to the patients".

The women disclosed their personal agonies and traumas. The following account is a reproduction of what was said in the group setting.

Have you ever taken any victim of violence to any health facility?

Specific responses

"Please don't ask this question," a participant voiced behind her veil.

"Yes." (Five respondents)

Which one?

"Myself", "*mein*." (Five respondents – two in an almost chorus style)

What was the type of violence?

"Badly beaten by my husband." (Five respondents)

Who attended the "victim"?

"A doctor and nurse."

How was the treatment?

"Very good and encouraging." (Sarcastic tone of a respondent)

What kind of treatment was given?

"A bandage and medicine because of severe swelling." (One respondent)

How do you rate this experience?

"It is different each time." (Three respondents)

Jamshoro district, Sindh

"*Ji waya ahiyon eelahi dafa bukhar, pet mein soor, bar beemar honda aahin ain asan pan beemar honda ahiyon par sarkari ispatlon jo karo monh aahiay.*" (Yes, we have been to government health facilities many times for abdominal cramps or other illness of our children or when we are ill ourselves – but the entire system of the health facilities in the public sector is distorted – it does not seem that human beings exist there.)

Use of any health facility and treatment options

The pattern for the women in Jamshoro is the same as that recorded in the focus group discussions with the women in Hyderabad. On the subject of contraception, they are of the opinion that although men support them in family planning, it is for women only "because they don't use any contraceptive and it would be used by us".

Health care for pregnant women

Again, the pattern for the women in Jamshoro is the same as that recorded in the focus group discussion with the women in Hyderabad. In addition, the women pointed out the use of Suzuki pick-ups and rented cars for transport when a pregnant or severely unwell woman has to be taken to a facility in the city or in Karachi.

Violence – general views

> "*Aurtoon ko Islam mein bhi kam samjha jata hay wo to paon ki joti hay jaisay chaho istamal karo.*" (Women are inferior even in Islam – they are like footwear – they can be used the way one wishes to.) (A woman respondent)

The pattern for the women in Jamshoro is again the same as that recorded in the focus group discussion with the women in Hyderabad. The commonest form of violence to them is the *watta satta/adla badla* (exchange marriages) and polygamy for heirs, especially sons.

> "*Betay ki aulad na honay ki waja say char char shadian karna.*" (If a son does not have any child or son, his parents go for even four marriages.)

Gender-based violence and health facilities

They have heard horrible stories of treatment of victims at the government hospitals but they themselves have no personal experience of taking any victim to, or seeing any victim in, any health facility.

However, when it comes to addressing the issues of domestic violence and abduction or assisting a girl who elopes or is raped, the respondents are of the view that health service providers are "nothing, because the police, jirga and community personalities will not hear them".

Muzaffarabad district, Azad Jammu and Kashmir

> "Can I register my complaint about day-to-day domestic violence that I face in my four walls. Both my mother-in-law and sister-in-law psychologically torture me as I have not brought with me a huge dowry at the time of my marriage. My parents were poor. My life is miserable and I want a normal and peaceful life – what can health providers do for me?" (A young woman respondent)

Use of any health facility and treatment options, and health care for pregnant women

The responses here are almost the same as those of the women from Hyderabad and Jamshoro. However, one new response was that they mentioned that they mostly walk to reach a health facility and use public transport as a second choice. Another new response was an emphasis on the changing attitudes of men towards contraception (which was also hinted at in the focus group discussions in Sindh) with the reservation that "religious-minded men don't allow themselves to do so".

Violence – general views

As in Sindh, the women were not familiar with the terms "gender-based violence/violence against women" in English or Urdu but when these terms were explained, they verified their prevalence, especially after the birth of daughters. Regarding home-based violence and sexual harassment in their area, they consider it a crime against innocent women and demand that it should be eliminated.

Specific responses

"It is quite commonly found in the lives of innocent Kashmiri women in its various shapes."

"Negligence and inadequate knowledge about their rights contribute towards violence in the lives of women."

"No involvement of women in decision-making, exercised by men only, is also violence against women."

"Violence means physical punishment and neglect by their men."

"It is visible especially where there is no education and awareness about their rights in rural areas, while in city areas it is low in average fortunately."

"It is getting reduced now as the media plays a pivotal role in spreading public messages about women rights."

"Yes, they face domestic violence; most of the women are not involved in decision-making powers at any level, and are not allowed to access modern medical health facilities and higher education."

If a woman is living in a violent relationship or has experienced violence, how might she get help?

The responses to this particular query are different from those in Sindh as they suggest some solutions or at least something more than just surrendering to the difficult circumstances.

Specific responses

"They get help from some of their sympathetic family members, both men and women, and also involve themselves in spirituality and religious practices."

"Weeping is a good catharsis and so are religious prayers and recitation of the Quran."

"Some of them also contact a psychiatrist or psychologist to get mental and psychological healing."

Gender-based violence and health facilities

General responses

Free medical treatment and a warm, friendly atmosphere are needed to address cases of violence against women at the health facility.

Specific responses

> "Responsible and professional staff with good attitudes and sound characters are needed but where are they?"

Expectations from different levels of health care facilities

Kashmiri women described in detail what they expect from different levels of health care facilities and providers.

Basic health units

These should be equipped with modern medical facilities, for example a medical laboratory, X-ray machines and ultrasound facilities. There should be a gynaecologist available 24 hours a day, along with medical officers and other staff.

Rural health centres

These should be established with basic health facilities at village level to be accessed by anyone at any time.

District headquarters hospitals

Medical officers should be highly qualified and demonstrate good behaviour with patients. Free medicine, free clinical tests and magnetic resonance imaging, ultrasound, etc., should be provided in each hospital. Gynaecologists, psychiatrists, psychologists, surgeons should be inducted.

Medical officers

They should be able to diagnose the nature of violence and treat the patient accordingly and should be able to provide counselling along with medical treatment.

Specialist doctors

They should raise awareness in the general population about gender-based violence through electronic, printed media and public messages. They should also inform victims about legal protection and treat these patients with special care.

Nurses

They should have adequate knowledge about gender-based violence and treat patients with special care, for example provide counselling, advice and guidelines.

Lady health visitors

They should treat the victims gently. As they serve at grass-roots level, they should also spread the message at village level to help eliminate the problem.

Lady health workers

They should also treat patients with great care and should raise awareness and campaign against gender-based violence.

Traditional birth assistants

They should preferably refer the victim to a specialist doctor, rather than treating them themselves. They should handle emergency cases carefully.

Kasur district, Punjab

Use of any health facility and treatment options, and health care for pregnant women

The responses were similar to those of the women from Sindh and Azad Jammu and Kashmir. One new response was that they emphasized the supportive attitudes of men towards them during pregnancy.

> "My husband treated me properly during my pregnancy, he even admitted me to a private hospital for proper treatment." (A young woman respondent)

Specific responses

> "No, they (men) are against family planning." (Responses of two participants from different age groups)

Violence – general views

General responses

Following an explanation of the terms "gender-based violence/violence against women" in Panjabi by the moderator, the women started a much more frank and fair discussion. There is a consensus that violence is a common fact in all Pakistani, including Kasur, women's lives.

They pointed out that husbands beat their wives not only with their bare hands but also with sticks and it is an open secret.

Specific responses

> "Due to frequent births of daughters, all the members of family have rude behaviour towards a woman."

> "Property issues are also becoming a source of violence against women."

Gender-based violence and health facilities

The respondents had no direct or indirect experience of taking a victim to a health facility. However, they stress the need to improve the standards of health facilities and availability of sympathetic staff. They are of the opinion that, other than traditional birth assistants, all health service providers such as medical doctors, lady health visitors and lady health workers can assist women victims when they are in need of medical help.

Profiles of the respondents from all eight focus group discussions are given in Annex 5.

Overall impressions from the focus group discussions

Gender-based violence is a living reality in all parts of Pakistan. Poverty and lack of education are offered as reasons to justify "wife battering" but these reasons can never legitimize brutal acts of violence.

The community, though poor, is well informed and enlightened, mainly due to the influx of television channels. However, changing lifestyles, as evident by the fact that even a poor person can afford a mobile phone, have failed to change the traditional patriarchal mindset where males remain the decision-makers in nearly all spheres of life.

Even today, sons are preferred, girls are verbally and physically abused on bringing a lesser dowry, and family planning is still considered un-Islamic and, if at any stage adopted, not with the intention of saving or improving a mother's life but only because of economic pressures.

Men are usually the perpetrators of violence but a number of cases of violence involve mothers-in-law. There are also men in the community who have the courage to condemn such practices openly and it can be hoped that they practice what they preach.

Urban-based communities, and even those in rural areas where access is possible, prefer to seek tertiary levels of health care.

Alternative sources of medical treatment are adopted, not because of any religious affinity, but mostly due to financial affordability and cultural access to such healers, who may be friendlier towards poor people, especially women.

Administrative snags in dealing with cases of violence cause immense trouble to the victim's supporters and bring a bad name to the community of doctors in particular, and all health service providers in general.

The invasion of television cameras in situations within a hospital setting worsens the situation and the person who suffers the most is the victim, who experiences physical injury, social pressures and mental trauma.

A rapid qualitative analysis based on the profiles of the focus group discussions (men and women) is given in Tables 3 and 4.

Table 3. A rapid qualitative analysis based on the profile of the focus group discussions (men).

Parameter	Area			
	Hyderabad	Jamshoro	Muzaffarabad	Kasur
Age range (years)	26–47	21–38	29–40	27–51
Education	Literate:illiterate 5:2	All educated	All literate	Literate:iilliterate 5:3
Marital status	Married:unmarried 6:1 The youngest in the group was single	Married:unmarried 4:2	All married	Married:unmarried 6:2
No. of children	The oldest in the group has highest number of alive children	More children for the oldest in the group	All with alive children	Oldest respondent with highest number of children
Employment status	All employed Public:private 2:5 More were employed in formal and informal private sector jobs, e.g. small shopkeepers	2 unemployed	All employed	1 unemployed
Access to television, mobile phone, radio, newspapers	In spite of belonging to what is perceived to be a low socioeconomic strata, all participants have access to television, mobile phones, radio (as owners) and newspapers (inaccessible only to the illiterate)	In spite of belonging to what is perceived to be a low socioeconomic strata, all participants have access to television, mobile phones, radio (as owners) and newspapers	In spite of belonging to what is perceived to be a low socioeconomic strata, all participants have access to television, mobile phones, radio (as owners) and newspapers	In spite of belonging to what is perceived to be a low socioeconomic strata, all participants have access to television, mobile phones, radio (as owners) and newspapers (inaccessible only to the illiterate)
Any disability	No physical or mental disability was evident or declared	No physical or mental disability was evident or declared	No physical or mental disability was evident or declared	No physical or mental disability was evident or declared

Table 4. A rapid qualitative analysis based on the profile of the focus group discussions (women).

Parameter	Area			
	Hyderabad	Jamshoro	Muzaffarabad	Kasur
Age range (years)	22–40	28–39	21–41	23–53
Education	All literate	Illiterate: literate 4:2	All literate	5 illiterate
Marital status	5 married	All married	7 married; Status undisclosed for one woman	One was unmarried and was also a student
No. of children	Oldest with more live children	More live children with more years in marriage	More children with more years in marriage	Oldest has the highest number of live children
Employment status	Work as housewife is not considered work; Paid workers have no control on their salaries	Work as housewife is not considered work; Paid workers have no control on their salaries (similar pattern as observed in Hyderabad, Sindh)	Work as housewife is not considered work; Paid workers have no control on their salaries (similar pattern as observed in Hyderabad and Jamshoro, Sindh)	Work as housewife is not considered work
Access to television, mobile phone, radio, newspapers	In spite of belonging to what is perceived and understood as the low socio-economic strata, all participants have access to television, mobile phones, radio) and newspaper(similar pattern as	In spite of belonging to what is perceived and understood as the low socio-economic strata, all participants have access to television, mobile phones, radio) and	In spite of belonging to what is perceived and understood as the low socio-economic strata, all participants have access to television, mobile phones, radio) and newspapers (similar pattern as observed in	In spite of belonging to what is perceived and understood as the low socio-economic strata, all participants have access to television) and with exception of 2, all have access to mobile phones; Only one had radio access (the single student)

	observed in Hyderabad Sindh)	newspaper (similar pattern as observed in Hyderabad Sindh)	Hyderabad and Jamshoro, Sindh)	
Any disability	No physical or mental disability was evident or declared	No physical or mental disability was evident or declared	No physical or mental disability was evident or declared	No physical or mental disability was evident or declared
Purdah[a] **observing/veiled**	Purdah:non-purdah 4:2 Suffering is same and veil does not act as protector or enhancer when it comes to violence This also points out that violence is also prevalent in families who are seen as religious; perhaps they are more into ritual actual teachings of religion that emphasize on a woman's right and non-violence are ignored, overlooked and forgotten	Purdah:non-purdah 4:2 Analysis is the same as for Hyderabad women	Purdah:non-purdah 3:4 Analysis is same as for Hyderabad and Jamshoro women in Sindh	Nobody was veiled but all were draped in chaddars/dupattas

[a] Purdah or pardaa (literally meaning "curtain") is the practice of preventing women from being seen by men. According to one definition, purdah is a curtain which makes sharp separation between the world of man and that of a woman, between the community as a whole and the family that is its heart, between the street and the home, the public and the private, just as it sharply separates society and the individual. This takes two forms: physical segregation of the sexes and the requirement for women to cover their bodies and conceal their form. Purdah exists in various forms in the Islamic world and among Hindu and Christian women in many parts of Pakistan.

Chapter 5. Findings and the way forward

This chapter assembles the findings and suggests some recommendations for the way forward to inform policy-makers for improved strategic planning and action for effective integration of gender-based violence into the health sector of Pakistan and Azad Jammu and Kashmir (the latter, however, also needs to be examined separately in the light of its different constitutional status).

Findings

General findings

The primary objective of the study was to assess the capacity of the health sector in Pakistan to integrate the issues of gender-based violence (interlinked, though not necessarily the same, concepts and terms are violence against women, girls and children) and this was done through a rapid assessment that employed qualitative methods.

While it is neither fair nor possible to document findings in statistical phrases or expressions using "high, moderate or less" grades, it is important and pertinent to describe the meanings of the measure.[52]

The scope of capacity development goes beyond the traditional donor focus on internal functioning of individual formal organizations, for example on their structures, systems, strategies, staff and skills (i.e. what might be termed the "micro" aspect of capacity development). The latest trend in result-based management is to look at the "macro" aspect, i.e. the behaviour and functioning of "work communities", particularly clusters of groups, organizations or individuals that deal with complex multifaceted functions such as environmental protection or rural health improvement.[53]

This assessment thus attempts to assess "capacity" in its different meanings and dimensions to address gender-based violence (Box 3).

---

[52] Capacity constraints are likely to stem not from a single cause (i.e. lack of skilled staff) but from a pattern or deeper structure of interlocking forces that combine to prevent system improvement. Attention to only one activity or part of the system (e.g. organizational restructuring) may have little impact at the broader system level. Cause and effect have a complex relationship separated by place, function and time. Dysfunctional behaviour inside an organization may have an explanation far outside the organization. Results "chains" are usually difficult to plot. Indicators do not explain why complex systems work the way they do (Morgan, 1997).
[53] Gender-based violence can also be included in the list.

Box 3. A checklist of different meanings and dimensions.

- Capacity to individually recognize issues of gender-based violence as a public health issue.
- Capacity to collectively recognize issues of gender-based violence as a public health issue.
- Capacity to respond to emerging issues of gender-based violence at the health facility level.
- Capacity to recognize the positive value of addressing gender-based violence.
- Capacity to initiate a change at the community level.
- Capacity to learn, i.e. the ability to respond to feedback in order to improve the quality of the action.
- Capacity to sustain, i.e. the ability to ensure continuity of action.
- Capacity to handle constraints, i.e. the ability to work with and use constraints.
- Capacity to maintain a programme, i.e. the ability to continue the routine effort required by a long-term programme.
- Capacity to adapt, i.e. the ability to integrate the innovative programme into the range of other programmes and processes in society.

Capacity indicators should not be based on the conventional "inputs–outputs outcomes–impact" typology that is widely used in the development community. They should focus more on process and behavioural change. Too many complex sets of indicators appear to be based on the flimsiest of change strategies. This strategy question is crucial to answering the "so what" question that applies to most indicators.[54]

The critical findings of the rapid assessment, taking into consideration the checklist in Box 3, are:

- Prevalence of gender-based violence in its various forms is higher in rural areas. However, the violence faced by urban lower- or middle-class women, including working women, and even by those within the health sector, needs to be explored.

- Characteristics of violence include: verbal abuse; physical abuse; hurting emotionally and physically; intimidating; isolation; control over personal things; humiliation; assault; neglect; threats to children and family; controlling social life, money and food; taking away liberty; substance abuse; and resisting self-expression.

- The health sector does not have any policy on addressing gender-based violence.

- The health systems are devoid of data management systems for gender-based violence.

- The health sector has almost no support mechanisms and intersectoral/multisectoral links with regard to gender-based violence.

- The links between disaster management, gender and health are also little understood and visibility cannot be determined.

---

[54] Source: Morgan (1997).

Findings as per the predetermined key areas of enquiry

Key barriers

The assessment found that health delivery staff face different types of barriers (e.g. social, political, administrative) in terms of attitudes and beliefs about violence against women while providing a health services.

Doctors face perceived and actual social barriers if they provide or attempt to provide assistance to victims of violence, who are usually women or young girls, as violence or domestic violence is considered to be a very private matter.

Religious leaders and some religious teachings have given rise to certain sociocultural factors that influence the health of women/girls and men/boys and affect the work of medical doctors and other health service providers.

Biases, perceptions and understanding of the health service provider

There are reasons, some of which are concealed, to explain the prevalence and characteristics of gender-based violence in the catchment areas of the different levels of health facilities.

Women and girls not only face various restrictions within the household but they are also less likely to access a health facility in time of need.

While boys and men enjoy freedom of mobility and can, if they so wish, access a health care facility more conveniently, even for minor ailments, women and girls are brought to a health facility only when they are quite unwell.

Women usually only consult health care providers for their children or when their disease has advanced and they can bear it no more. One common example is that of tuberculosis, when women tend to hide due to the fear of the shame and stigma associated with this disease.

As far as health-seeking behaviour is concerned, this varies between urban and rural population and there is no gender-based specification. Rural dwellers tend to visit government facilities because medicines, if available, are free of cost in those service points. Urban dwellers also visit hospitals in the public sector but they prefer private clinics.

Existing capacities of respondents to identify hidden symptoms of gender-based violence and whether they are aware of and refer survivors of gender-based violence to local psychosocial services

In the health sector, all health service providers have a role in addressing gender-based violence. Unfortunately, there are no counsellor posts in the public sector. As psychosocial counselling is necessary for victims of gender-based violence, either a new position should be created or lady health workers and lady health visitors should be given financial incentives to train as counsellors.

One advantage of being a health provider is that people generally have a lot of faith in them and have respect for them and hence they are in a good position to detect and resolve issues of gender-based violence.

Healthcare professionals tend to consider cases of gender-based violence as medico-legal; they are scared of becoming involved in this subject and limit themselves to treating the physical injuries.

There is clear evidence that gender-based violence is a preventable public health problem. However, despite the increasing evidence of the serious health consequences of gender-based violence, health systems in many countries, including Pakistan, are not fully geared towards addressing the issues. Several studies show that health professionals in many countries have not received training or professional development on gender-based violence and responding to violence is not seen as part of their role.

Support mechanisms and existing resources for health care providers to address cases of gender-based violence

There are virtually no support mechanisms that are sufficient to integrate gender-based violence into the health sector.

Existing health sector capacities and links with other sectors/line departments/civil society organizations to identify and address gender-based violence; sensitive ways of communicating with patients about gender-based violence; responding to and documenting cases of gender-based violence

These capacities have already been discussed under general findings. Existing capacities are at a very embryonic level and a number of multi-coordinated efforts are required to build and sustain the required capacities.

Health sector structural readiness to address gender-based violence

The following issues need to be addressed:

- levels of privacy in health centres, effective sound barriers, effective visual barriers;
- storage of, and access to, medical records;
- capacity to maintain privacy and confidentiality;
- referral to, and awareness of, available resources/support (e.g. medical care; medico-legal information);
- capacity and resources available for recording cases of gender-based violence.

While the infrastructure of the health care facilities permits privacy, the concepts of privacy and confidentiality are not translated into actual practice.

Health service providers and decision-makers:

- are largely driven by the same attitudes, beliefs and laws that are prevalent in society and these are, regretfully, anti-women and against socially disadvantaged women and men in Pakistan;
- are, to a large extent, unsure or unconvinced of the role of health care providers in addressing gender-based violence and its relevance to the health sector;

- need to understand the relevance of health, gender and gender-based violence, as there are gaps in their understanding of the basics;
- need to concentrate on improving the communication skills of clinicians and health workers in relation to gender-based violence;
- need to have a clear and consistent understanding of gender issues and health needs of the different sexes and age groups;
- need to understand very clearly the social and health outcomes of gender-based violence; for example, HIV/AIDS issues need to be understood by health service providers as no one mentioned these in any context in the study.

Challenges and conclusions

Attitudes and beliefs

In the light of the reviewed literature, respondents' narratives and field observations, the key barriers faced by health delivery staff in terms of attitudes and beliefs about violence against women can be grouped into four categories: administrative, technical capacity, community and society.

Administrative

Administrative challenges include:

- lack of sensitivity towards issues of gender-based violence and apathy of policy-level officials to address these issues in the health services;
- lack of leadership for these issues in the health services;
- lack of services required to deal with gender-based violence;
- lack of monitoring of issues of gender-based violence by health services;
- lack of knowledge;
- lack of commitment;
- exclusion of duties and actions related to gender-based violence in the terms of reference or job descriptions of heath service providers.

Technical capacity

Technical capacity challenges include:

- lack of training, thus limited capacity, on issues of gender-based violence;
- limited knowledge among health service providers about issues of gender-based violence.

Community

Community challenges include:

- lack of community support for issues of gender-based violence;

- cultural barriers within the community;
- illiteracy;
- poor communication between husbands and wives;
- joint family systems (in some cases);
- abject poverty;
- geographic inaccessibility;
- acceptance of violence against women as routine or the norm.

Society

Challenges within society include:

- cultural barriers;
- the conservatism of relatives and women themselves;
- superstitious minds that accept violence as their fate and therefore do not accept help; women may also resist help as they will then have to reveal the person responsible for their condition.

Health service providers' perceptions and understanding of gender-based violence; its causes, prevalence, characteristics and impact on health services

Perceptions

Perceptions include:

- violence is part of life;
- women deserve violence to some extent;
- it is not a big issue;
- gender-based violence is characterized by health care professionals as an extremely difficult problem and is not generally accounted for in diagnoses, although physical injuries, headache, digestive problems, sexual dysfunction, depression and hypertension are common;
- health care professionals tend to consider cases of gender-based violence as more pertinent to medico-legal fields and are scared of becoming involved in this subject thus limit themselves to treating the physical injuries.

Understanding

Understanding includes:

- gender-based violence is prevalent worldwide but developing countries are especially hard hit;

- gender-based violence is related to organic diseases such as HIV and other sexually transmitted diseases;
- gender-based violence is intimately related to illiteracy and lack of empowerment of women.

Health service providers do not understand jargon such as "gender" or "gender-based violence/violence against women and girls" but they understand the common forms of this violence and recognize the signs, especially obvious physical injuries. History-taking on sexual assaults and domestic violence is a difficult area and they may miss internal injuries in an overcrowded clinic, or in some cases they may not be competent in diagnosis.

Reasons for gender-based violence

Reasons for violence at the household and community levels include:

- domestic disharmony;
- illiteracy;
- economic instability;
- psychosocial problems;
- drugs;
- cultural values;
- non-acceptance of the issue (a tendency to discuss domestic violence as something that only happened to others);
- situational and economically driven early marriages (e.g. the traditional practice of *watta satta*).

Health sector institutions are not ready to integrate gender-based violence into their existing systems. The following factors exacerbate gender-based violence and weaken institutional capacity to integrate these issues into public health systems:

- uncertain donor support and international commitment;
- media interference;
- lack of assistance and protection by the Government.

Support mechanisms and resources for health care providers to address gender-based violence

Resources are available to address gender-based violence but there is a strong and immediate need to develop the capacities of various cadres of policy-makers or professionals to increase their sensitivity to, and acceptance of, these issues.

There is a specific need for:

- utilization of the available infrastructure;

- review of health policy and strategic plans;
- appropriate allocation of budget from available financial resources;
- sensitization of health service providers;
- capacity-building and technical training;
- establishing a support system that guarantees sustained links not only within the health sector but also outside it, i.e. with allied line departments and organizations.

Links with other sectors, line departments and organizations

There are at present no links with other sectors/line departments/civil society organizations to address gender-based violence. The lack of staff, deficient skills and absence of motivation is evidence of this. Anti-women beliefs and attitudes and non-liberal thinking are evident within certain sections of health service providers and there are many inherent weaknesses of the health system within the larger bureaucratic apparatus.

However, half-hearted efforts have been made to create links with the following sectors:

- education, to improve literacy;
- the media;
- the judiciary;
- economic empowerment;
- psychological counselling centres.

Awareness of any national policies or laws that exist to prevent gender-based violence and awareness of laws or policies that require specific actions by health service providers with regard to these issues is lacking. According to some, laws have even been made to the contrary. Nearly all the experts are unaware of any laws and policies for women and for health service providers, except for medico-legal procedures. However, some respondents did mention the anti-harassment at the workplace law that was enforced by the Government in 2010.

Strengths and weaknesses of the health sector's structural readiness to address gender-based violence

One of the key conclusions is the identification of factors within the health sector that determine its strengths and weaknesses to address issues surrounding gender-based violence.

The health sector's strengths are:

- availability of human resources;
- good opportunities to deal with gender-based violence;
- its interdepartmental links;
- the willingness of the administrative staff;

- its presence at the grass-roots level.

Its weakness are:

- an absence of well-defined policies on gender-based violence;
- an absence of commitment against gender-based violence;
- the lack of commitment of staff towards work due to a variety of factors;
- cultural non-acceptance of gender equality;
- the friction between nongovernmental organizations and public sector workers at individual and departmental levels;
- non-functional support systems;
- lack of understanding of the complexity of issues of gender-based violence.

Policy recommendations for the health sector

Integration at policy level

In its 49th Assembly, WHO declared gender-based violence a global public health emergency. The first and foremost follow-up action should be the recognition of gender-based violence as a public health issue and its integration into the country's health policy. Furthermore, its inclusion must be articulated in a very loud and clear way that strongly encourages the political will and readiness of the bureaucratic apparatus to accept and endorse the integration. In Pakistan, even well-articulated, progressive and inclusive policies fall prey to ineffective implementation.

The Ministry of Health is being closed down in a few months, and provinces will become responsible for delivery on health. It is strongly urged that the capacities of the provinces are developed to effectively deliver integration of gender-based violence, in particular its specific integration into the provincial health service, preferably supervised by a female district health officer (currently nearly all are men) at the district level.

Policy-makers must approve guidelines and protocols for standard treatment of women victims of violence and these must be disseminated not only in English but also in Urdu, Pashto, Sindhi and other local languages at all levels of health care facilities.

Capacity-building of health service providers to address issues of gender-based violence

As an important step towards the prevention of gender-based violence, a supportive, violence-aware practice environment should be provided, where health service providers use sympathetic and empowering language that is appropriate to each patient, know how to conduct a physical examination to confirm physical/sexual assault and are aware of local services to which abused women can be referred.

It is also very important that health service providers know how to provide thorough treatment, not only for the physical consequences of abuse but also for its mental health ramifications, including post-traumatic stress disorder.

Physicians and other health care providers should look on the treatment of abused women as a complicated and multidimensional clinical problem and provide specific practical suggestions and resources relevant to the continuum of care, from diagnosis and immediate intervention to long-term management. To meet such standards, the capacity of not only doctors but also other health care professionals, paramedics and the entire administrative machinery needs to be built up. This exercise must be preceded by careful research that clearly identifies capacity gaps, training needs and the essential set of information, knowledge and skills that should be imparted. It must be emphasized that attitudinal and behavioural change exercises must be embedded within such training.

Some suggested areas of training, which are by no means comprehensive, are given in Box 4.

Box 4. Suggested areas of training.

Empathy
Perceptions and understanding of gender: essential concepts
Health staff attitudes; acknowledging biases within health service providers; becoming non-judgemental
Forms of gender-based violence
Ability to identify hidden symptoms of gender-based violence and clinical management
Medical jurisprudence (for doctors and executive district officers/district health officers)
Communication skills (with community, clients, victims, perpetrators)
Knowledge about existing support mechanisms, laws to protect women and links
Definitions of youth and adolescent and their specific health needs
History-taking skills
Psychosocial counselling skills
Assertive negotiation skills (to be conveyed to the victims)
Survivor-centred approach
Engaging men in ending violence against women
Record keeping and data management

Gender-based violence and disasters[55]

The burden of disaster, like the burden of disease, is higher for women and there is a lack of a gender perspective in disaster preparedness and management, both at policy planning and design level. However, even though it is said that women suffer disproportionately, it does not mean that all women suffer more than men or that their experiences are necessarily similar to one another. Like men, women are not a homogenous group. It is strongly recommended that due attention and acknowledgement is given to increased gender-based violence in disaster scenarios as it directly impacts on health of women, children and men.

Specific practical action

Global programme experience suggests that training health care providers and raising awareness about gender-based violence may not be enough. Rather, to support women survivors of violence, entire health systems need to respond, with links to legal and social services. The following actions are required:

- Revamping the weaknesses of the medico-legal system, from undergraduate studies to practice, to make it more professional. This will require extensive consultation with duty bearers and stakeholders who are involved as curriculum experts, examiners and decision-makers for graduate and postgraduate medical education and administration.[56]

- There is also a need to further examine alternative measures for enhancing justice for victims of sexual assault. An important question to be answered is: how might such measures be prioritized in terms of resource allocation vis-à-vis existing criminal justice and medico-legal practices?[57]

- There are several laws that protect women from violence but awareness of these is low and their enforcement is weak. Effective dissemination of information on gender-based violence through all channels of communication is required.

---

[55] This assessment did not focus on the capacity of the health sector to respond to gender-based violence in disasters like floods and in conflict settings but these are vital considerations and must be included and integrated at policy and programme levels.

[56] "When medico-legal examinations are performed, they are frequently conducted in a haphazard manner and fail to secure meaningful evidence. Doctors focus on determining whether and when the hymen was broken rather than on collecting evidence to demonstrate the extent and severity of women's injuries and to identify offenders. In some cases, unmarried women who, in the examining doctors' opinion, were not virgins prior to being attacked, tend to be harassed and their rape allegations disbelieved by the doctors. The examination findings also render them vulnerable to attacks on their character by defence counsel and, potentially, to prosecution for prior illicit sex. The focus on the hymen also militates against effective examinations of sexually active married women because their injuries are not usually related to hymenal tearing. In addition to shoddy examinations, chemical analysis of forensic samples collected from the examinees is commonly mishandled, and produces unreliable results." Excerpt from a report by Burney (1999) that follows a 1992 report, *Double jeopardy: Police abuse of women in Pakistan*, which documented sexual abuse of women by state agents.

[57] Borrowed from a review commissioned by WHO for the Sexual Violence Research Initiative, an international initiative supported by the Global Forum for Health Research, as it is equally valid in Pakistan-specific context (Du Mont & White, 2008).

- Women's neighbourhood self-help groups could be an effective, socially relevant and sustainable agency to prevent local violence (in the garb of, say, "safe women, healthy, happy families").
- Active involvement of key stakeholders, effective players and civil society representatives in developing ownership of issues surrounding gender-based violence and violence against women, girls and children.
- Active involvement of related government line departments at various levels with clear and viable interventions/plans of action for gender-based violence.
- Prompt justice for the victims through establishing the required systems of procedures and coordination.
- Specific measures are needed to develop health service providers' awareness of HIV/AIDS issues, as no-one mentioned these in any context in the study.
- Introduction of a survivor-centred approach in programme management within the health sector to address issues of gender-based violence.

Using global experiences to learn how to improve issues of gender-based violence in the health sector is one critical step forward. Some key recommendations documented in the literature for improve the capacity and response of the health sector regarding gender-based violence are as follows:[58]

- addressing gender-based violence calls for a systemic health sector approach;
- building political will and ensuring allocation of adequate resources to address gender-based violence;
- embarking on a gender-sensitive coordinated system-wide approach linking local, regional and international mechanisms to prevent, monitor and manage gender-based violence;
- integrating selective or comprehensive services for victims of gender-based violence into primary, secondary and tertiary care, as part of overall or selective health care services, especially sexual and reproductive health, including adolescent health, antenatal care, postnatal care, family planning and HIV/AIDS/sexually transmitted infections; child health care; emergency medicine; mental and psychosocial health; ear, nose and throat care; and dental care.
- building a health infrastructure with adequate security and private examination and counselling rooms;
- clarifying providers' roles, including education and training in gender-based violence, into the pre- and post-service training of health personnel;
- having gender-sensitive services;
- including males in sexual and reproductive health and childcare, not only as providers, but as true partners;
- ensuring primary prevention;

---

[58] Source: *Gender-based violence, health and the role of the health sector* (http://web.worldbank.org/WBSITE/EXTERNAL/TOPICS/EXTHEALTHNUTRITIONANDPOPULATION/EXTPHAAG/0,,contentMDK:22421973~pagePK:64229817~piPK:64229743~theSitePK:672263,00.html, accessed November 2010).

- rehabilitating and managing chronic conditions.

Improve quality of care for survivors of gender-based violence and others

To improve quality of care the following are recommended:

- sensitize, educate, train, supervise, support and monitor health personnel to improve knowledge, attitudes and practices regarding gender-based violence;
- develop, introduce and monitor management protocols and guidelines for gender-based violence;
- screen to ensure early diagnosis and intervention as an integrated part of reproductive and sexual health services, as well as in other parts of the health sector and when physical injuries, health conditions and client behaviour raise the suspicion; emotional support and counselling – listen with respect to the survivor and acknowledge her autonomy;
- personal examination and routine enquiry in privacy, ensuring confidentiality and adequate registration;
- treatment and management of victims of gender-based violence, including testing, postexposure treatment and counselling on HIV/AIDS/sexually transmitted infections, pregnancy and emergency contraception; referral to legal social and community services in recognition of the need for safety, legal justice and social services;
- community-based care with early identification and support to victims of gender-based violence and their families;
- forensic examinations;
- gender-sensitive information, education and communication, including boys and men, targeting children and young people;
- addressing societal and cultural norms underlying gender-based violence to create increased public awareness of gender inequities, gender-based violence and the human rights of women and children;
- informing and educating civil servants, teachers, police, lawyers, social workers, public media and others on gender-based violence; mass media education/entertainment programmes.

Improve data collection, research and knowledge sharing on gender-based violence

To improve data collection, research and knowledge sharing, the following are recommended:

- strengthening medical and health information record-keeping, documentation and confidentiality in gender-based violence; including gender-based violence in demographic and household surveys; building local, national and international research capacity for knowledge collection and management to inform and advocate for policy reforms in the area of gender-based violence and monitoring the effectiveness and efficiency of interventions.

Strengthen intersectoral links with other ministries, civil society, nongovernmental organizations and the private sector to enhance awareness, prevent, monitor and manage gender-based violence

Effective community and society interventions are based on coordination between the legal, social, health and education system and the workplace (Bott, Morrison & Ellsberg, 2005). This is often furthered through decentralization:

- social services: shelters, child protection, income generating activities, community support and women's groups;
- education: involve the education system in the prevention and management of gender-based violence through promoting greater respect for girls and women and human rights as well as non-violence; enhance school safety (safe latrines for girls); school health education and school health; include education on gender-based violence in the higher education of health care providers, lawyers, social workers, teachers, police, etc.;
- legal: build alliance with the legal system to enhance enforcement of laws related to gender-based violence.

It is clear that the need for formative research to develop better and clearer understanding of local and indigenous perspectives, issues and priorities on the complex issues of gender-based violence remains of utmost importance.

All recommendations, if considered practically, would contribute towards new learning and improvements in the sector and set a standard of recommended practices to address gender-based violence, both in development and in disaster strategies.

Annex 1. Interview guide for health service providers in the public sector

Integrating response to violence in the health services[59]

Introduction

The purpose of the study is to evaluate the existing capacity of the health sector and the community to respond to gender-based violence/violence against women and girls[60] in the lives of clients or patients (boys, girls, men and women), pregnant mothers attending antenatal care and to women in the community at large.

Instructions for using the instrument

As usual with an in-depth discussion, the interviewers should ensure that the meeting is held in a comfortable space, that there will be no interruption and that there is some refreshment (at least water) available to the informants.

The interviewers should introduce themselves and establish rapport. Begin with an explanation of the purpose of the interview, benefits to the interviewees and intended uses of the information (e.g. "We are collecting baseline information on detection of gender-based violence, management practices that exist in the health facilities and your perceptions of your own and the facility's readiness to offer services related to gender-based violence"). State the number of questions and the approximate time it will take to complete the discussion.

Assure informants that the information collected here will be treated confidentially and that their names will not be used at all. In that light, encourage respondents to be honest and frank in their response to the questions asked.

The data collectors must get the informed verbal consent statement from all the respondents.

One person will be leading the interview while two others will take notes. In addition, if participants agree, the interview will be tape-recorded.

A guide can only serve as a general protocol for the interview. Issues may arise that were not foreseen in advance; indeed this is part of the value of interviewing rather than asking people to complete questionnaires. The interviewer should follow up on relevant topics that are raised by the informants.

---

[59] This questionnaire for the health service providers and the focus group discussions drew its inspiration from IntraHealth International (2008). The original document is licensed under the Creative Commons Attribution-Noncommercial-Share Alike 3.0 Licence. More information on this licence is available at: http://creativecommons.org/licenses/by-nc-sa/3.0/us, accessed November 2010.

[60] Gender-based violence and violence against women and girls have been used interchangeably in the document and, where needed, the distinction is highlighted.

At the end of the interview, thank the respondents for participating/rendering their views and restate the purpose and benefits of the study.

Consent

We are working on an assessment approved by WHO and an ethical review team. We want to talk to men/women who visit health service delivery points such as basic health units, rural health centres, district headquarters or tehsil headquarters.

The purpose of the study is to evaluate the capacity of the health sector and the community to respond to gender-based violence, for instance in the lives of clients and patients (boys, girls, men and women), pregnant mothers attending antenatal care and to women in the community at large.

We would like to ask you some questions to get information necessary to develop and monitor a health programme in support of women who live with violence, including pregnant women who use antenatal care services.

You will not be contacted in the future. We will not ask you for your name. Your answers are confidential and cannot be linked back to you. The questionnaires/tape recordings will be kept in a locked cabinet at the office of WHO Pakistan in Islamabad.

The only people who will see the questionnaires/tape recordings are people who are working on this study and who are strictly required to keep professional secrecy. Some people feel anxious or embarrassed when asked questions about their behaviour. Your participation is completely voluntary and you may decline to answer any specific question or completely refuse to participate.

We would greatly appreciate your help in responding to these questions, even though we are not able to financially compensate you. You may not personally or immediately benefit from this assessment, but the results will be used to improve health services for all citizens who use public sector health facilities.

The interview will take up to 40–50 minutes. If you have any questions, you can ask now, at any point during discussion or at the end of the session.

May we begin?

General information

Date (dd/mm/yy) _____/_____/_____ Start time _____ a.m./p.m.

Interviewers' names:

Last_____, First_____

Last_____, First_____

Facility information:

Name:

Address:

Language/s used:

Respondent (health service provider profile):[61]

Qualification:

No. of years of service:

No. of trainings received on gender:

No. of trainings received on gender-based violence/violence against women and girls:

No. of trainings received on gender and health:

No. of trainings received on any topic related to the health sector:

Kindly specify the name, theme/topic, duration and location of the training.

The questionnaire

Ice breakers:

Objectives:

Perceptions and understanding of respondents:

1. Have you heard of the word gender/*sinf*? Any idea? Any interpretation?

2. Is there any difference between sex and gender? Any idea? Please explain?

3. How common an experience do you think violence is in the

---

[61] To be filled out at the end of the interview.

lives of women in Pakistan?

4. How common an experience do you think violence is in the lives of women in your district/city/tehsil?

5. What types of violence have you heard or seen?

   Heard:

   Seen:

6. What are the common causes of violence against women and girls (e.g. dowry-related, marriage-related, doubts about a woman/girls' conduct, property disputes, son preference, differences with in-laws, schooling of girls, etc.)?

7. Do you think women and girls face any form of violence from your list here?

SECTION A: GENDER-BASED VIOLENCE AND HEALTH-RELATED CONSIDERATIONS

Objectives:

Key barriers faced by the health delivery staff in terms of attitudes and beliefs about gender-based violence/violence against women and girls while providing health services

8. Do you think you would face any barriers to address gender-based violence/violence against women and girls as health service provider?

   Yes:

   No:

   If yes, kindly identify:

9. Would you like to identify key sociocultural factors that influence health of women/girls and men/boys in your area of work (e.g. dowry-related, marriage-related, doubts about a woman/girls' conduct, property disputes,

   Women/girls:

   Men/boys:

	son preference, differences with in-laws, schooling of girls, etc.)?	
10.	Would you like to identify key biological factors that influence the health of women/girls and men/boys in your area of work?	Women: Girls: Boys: Men:
11.	Who can access and use health facility services easily?	Women/girls: Boys/men:
12.	What is the health-seeking behaviour of women/girls and boys/men?	Women/girls: Boys/men:
13.	What are the treatment options for women/girls and boys/men	Women/girls: Boys/men:
14.	What is your experience in health care settings with women/girls and boys/men? (Highlight some regarding violence)	Women/girls: Boys/men:
15.	Would you like to identify certain health and social outcomes and consequences of negligence of health considerations for women/girls and boys/men?	Women/girls: Boys/men:

SECTION B: REPORTED GENDER-BASED VIOLENCE RELATED EXPERIENCE

Objectives:

Existing capacities/actions of respondents to identify hidden symptoms of gender-based violence (physical, psychological and sexual abuse by intimate partners, in-laws and perpetrators), and whether they are aware of, and refer survivors of gender-based violence to, local psychosocial services

16. Who are your clients and patients?   Clients: Patients:

17. Have you ever worked with clients/patients who may have been victims of violence?

18. What has been your experience in working with clients/patients who may have been victims of violence?

19. Do you think health service providers who suspect that a client/patient was a victim of conjugal or sexual violence would usually ask their client/patient about it? What are the advantages or disadvantages to this?

20. Do you believe you could help a woman who was a victim of violence? Why or why not? If so, how?

21. Do you believe you could help a minor girl who was a victim of violence? Why or why not? If so, how?

22. Do you believe you could help a minor boy who was a victim of violence? Why or why not? If so, how?

23. Do you believe you could help another person who was a victim of violence? Why or why not? If so, how?

24. Do you refer cases of violence? Where? To whom?

    If not, why not (e.g. no such cases come to your health facility, you cannot recognize such cases or other reasons such as fears, pressures, duty/business rules)?

25. What usually happens when a woman comes into a health facility with injuries/disabilities or after a rape/sexual abuses? What kind of violence-related services would she find? What type of health service provider would assist her?

26. How are health service providers allowed to treat a victim of conjugal violence? Are they allowed to do the following:

Document injuries for legal cases?

Keep documentation confidential?

Any other?

SECTION C: INTEGRATION OF SERVICES FOR GENDER-BASED VIOLENCE

We are interested in how to integrate services for gender-based violence into health service provision.

Objectives:

Support mechanisms and existing resources for health care providers/delivery staff to address cases of gender-based violence, including presence of female health care providers; equipment/instruments; mechanisms for self-protection; relevant trainings/skills; communication channels.

Existing health sector capacities and links with other sectors/line departments/civil society organizations to address gender-based violence, including identifying gender-based violence, sensitive way of communicating with patients on gender-based violence (capacity to engage victims in conversation), responding to and documenting cases of gender-based violence

27. How is conjugal/domestic violence or another form (specify) currently addressed within a facility?

28. What services should be provided at an antenatal care centre related to conjugal violence/domestic violence/dowry violence?

29. Do you think that a client who uses antenatal care services might be at risk for any of the types of violence mentioned before? What types of violence? When might she experience this?

30. What services would be needed in order to address conjugal violence and other forms of violence?

31. What would be the role of the following:

    (a) nurses: (a)

    (b) physicians: (b)

    (c) counsellors: (c)

(d) lady health visitors: (d)

(e) lady health workers: (e)

32. Is the record-keeping system equipped to register and monitor incidents of gender-based violence?

    Who can access records/reports?

SECTION D: GENDER-BASED VIOLENCE, THE HEALTH SECTOR AND THE POST-FLOOD SCENARIO

33. Did you notice any incidence of gender-based violence/violence against women and girls during and after the floods? If "Yes", what form of violence and can you specify where?

    How are you treating or responding to these cases?

    Form of violence:

    Location:

    Other details:

34. Do you think the health sector is prepared to manage half a million pregnant women who are affected by floods?

35. Do you think the health sector is prepared to address the needs (kindly specify the needs) of flood-affected neonates, infants and children?

    Needs of neonates:

    Needs of infants:

    Needs of children (under 18 years):

36. Do you think the health sector is prepared to address the

    Adolescent girls (9–19 years):

needs (kindly specify the needs) of flood-affected adolescents and youth?

Adolescent boys (9–19 years):

Young girls (15 to 29 years):

Young boys (15–29 years):

37. Is the record-keeping system equipped to register and monitor incidents of gender-based violence?

    Who can access records?

38. What are the support mechanisms and existing resources for health care providers to address cases of gender-based violence, including presence of female health care providers, self-safety mechanisms, skills and communication channels?

39. What are the existing health sector capacities and links with other sectors/line departments/civil society organizations to address gender-based violence, including identifying gender-based violence, sensitive ways of communicating with patients on gender-based violence (e.g. capacity to engage victims in conversation), responding to and documenting cases of gender-based violence?

SECTION E: GENDER-BASED VIOLENCE AND THE MEDICO-LEGAL SYSTEM

40. Are you aware of national policies or laws that exist to prevent violence against women? If yes, which ones?

41. Are you aware of laws or policies that require specific actions by health service providers with regard to violence against women?

42. What role should the Government play in trying to address the problem of violence against women?

CHALLENGES AND RECOMMENDATIONS

43. Challenges and recommendations for improving health response (identification, screening, management and recording) to cases of gender-based violence

THANK YOU VERY MUCH!

[Time of end of interview: _____ a.m./p.m.]

Interview guide for the focus group discussions with men and women (in separate groups), who are the consumers of health services in the public sector

Consent

We are working on an assessment approved by WHO and an ethical review team. We want to talk to men/women who visit health service delivery points such as basic health units, rural health centres, and district headquarter or tehsil headquarter hospitals.

The purpose of the study is to evaluate the capacity of the health sector and the community to respond to gender-based violence in the lives of clients or patients (boys, girls, men and women), pregnant mothers attending antenatal care and to women in the community at large.

We would like to ask you some questions to get the information necessary to develop and monitor a health programme in support of women who live with violence, including pregnant women who use antenatal care services.

You will not be contacted in the future. We will not ask you for your name. Your answers are confidential and cannot be linked back to you. The questionnaires/tape recordings will be kept in a locked cabinet at the office of WHO Pakistan in Islamabad.

The only people who will see the questionnaires/tape recordings are people who are working on this study and who are strictly required to keep professional secrecy. Some people feel anxious or embarrassed when asked questions about their behaviour. Your participation is completely voluntary and you may decline to answer any specific question or completely refuse to participate.

We would greatly appreciate your help in responding to these questions, even though we are not able to financially compensate you. You may not personally or immediately benefit from this assessment, but the results will be used to improve health services for all citizens who use public sector health facilities.

The interview will take up to 60–90 minutes. If you have any questions, you can ask now, at any point during discussion or at the end of the session.

May we begin?

General information

Date (dd/mm/yy) _____/_____/_____ Start time _____ a.m./p.m.

Moderator's name:

Last_____, First_____

Note-takers' names:

Last_____, First_____

Last_____, First_____

Venue of the focus group discussion:

Name:

Address:

Language/s in which the discussion was conducted:

Number of respondents and personal details

Parameters	Respondent							
	1	2	3	4	5	6	7	8
Age (years)								
Education								
Marital status and no. of children								
Employment status								
Access to television								
Access to mobile phone								
Access to radio								
Access to newspaper								
Any disability								
Any other attribute								
Purdah observing/veiled (for women)								

Ice breakers

Inquire about their well-being and especially how they are doing after the floods.

Opening questions

How often do you visit any public sector health facility? Why?

What means of transport do you use? If you walk, then how many kilometres (approximately)?

Do you prefer a medical doctor or others such as traditional healers, homeopaths/etc.? If you answered "Yes", why?

Violence – general views

Do men support women in accessing health care during pregnancy?

Do men support women in accessing family planning services?

Have you ever heard the terminology "gender-based violence/violence against women"? (If not, the moderator will explain.)

What is your idea/concept of gender-based violence/violence against women?

How common an experience do you think violence is in the lives of women in Pakistan?

How common an experience do you think violence is in the lives of women in your district/city?

What types of violence have you heard or seen?

Do you think women and girls face any form of violence from your list here?

If a woman is living in a violent relationship or has experienced violence, how might she get help?

Gender-based violence/violence against women and health facilities

Have you ever taken any victim of violence to any health facility?

Which one?

What was the type of violence?

Who attended the victim?

How was the treatment?

What kind of treatment was given?

How do you rate this experience?

Experience sharing: tell a story (yours or that of someone else you know)

The moderator will request that respondents share any story of violence that they may have and describe their experience, in particular the connection with health service providers in the public sector.

Recommendations

What would your recommendations be to improve the services and standards of:

- Basic health units?
- Rural health centres?
- Tehsil headquarters?

- District headquarters?

How do you think the following health service providers can respond to cases of gender-based violence/violence against women:

- Medical officers?
- Specialist doctors?
- Nurses?
- Lady health visitors?
- Lady health workers?
- Counsellors?
- Traditional birth assistants?

Observations

The health sector's structural readiness to address gender-based violence will be observed through:

- attitudes, sensitivity, fears of health service providers at facilities to help survivors of gender-based violence and to address this issue as a health problem;
- levels of privacy in health centres, effective sound barriers, effective visual barriers;
- how medical records are stored and who has access to them;
- capacity to maintain privacy and confidentiality;
- referral (and awareness of) to available resources/support (medical care; medico-legal information);
- capacity and resources available for consistent recording of cases of gender-based violence.

Questions or health service providers who attended the training courses

What are the level and effectiveness of links between gender-based violence and health-related:

- Policies?
- Laws?
- Operational plans?
- Guidelines?

Annex 2. List of respondents

Health service providers who were interviewed and gave consent to disclose names

Hyderabad, Sindh

- Dr Anila Sammo (Woman Medical Officer)
- Dr Naseer Ahmed (Senior Medical Superintendent)
- Ms Ershad Sammo (Lady Health Visitor)
- Ms Shama Khaskheli (Lady Health Worker)
- Dr Bux Pitafi (Executive District Officer Health)

Jamshoro, Sindh

- Dr Niaz Abro (Medical Officer)
- Dr Anjum Sheikh (Woman Medical Officer)
- Dr Ali Abbas Khoso (Tehsil Headquarters Health Officer)

Muzaffarabad, Azad Jammu and Kashmir

- Ms Naheed Shah (Lady Health Visitor)
- Dr Shabbir Dar (Deputy Director Administration Department of Health)
- Dr Sabir Abbasi (District Health Officer)

Kasur, Punjab

- Dr Ijaz Sindhu (Family Planning Programme)
- Ms Shamim Akhter (Lady Health Worker)
- Ms Azmat Mansoor (Lady Health Visitor Supervisor and Trainer)
- Dr Khalid Rhandawa (Executive District Officer Health)
- Dr Muhammad Shakoor (District Health Officer)

Health service providers who participated in the group discussion

Jamshoro, Sindh

- Dr Shahidah Memon (Senior Trainer)
- Ms Gulzar Sammo (Lady Health Worker)
- Ms Shabana Somro (Lady Health Visitor)
- Dr Deedar Ali (Chief Medical Officer)

- Dr Nisar Ahmed Bughio (Chief Medical Officer)
- Dr Ghulam Qadir Nareejo (Deputy Tehsil Health Officer in Executive District Office)

Muzaffarabad, Azad Jammu and Kashmir

- Mr Fazal Husain Awan (Office Assistant, Basic Development Needs Programme)
- Mr Mukhtar Awan (Programme Manager, Basic Development Needs Programme)
- Mr Khawaja Yasir (Community Mobilizer, Basic Development Needs Programme)
- Mr Raja Abdullah Khan (Chairman, Basic Development Needs Programme)
- Ms Rukhsana Awan (Assistant Director, Shaheed Benazir Bhutto Women Development Centre)
- Ms Nilofer Faiz (Project Officer, Basic Development Needs Programme)
- Mr Khawajia Fiaz Ahmed (Finance Assistant, Basic Development Needs Programme)

Kasur, Azad Jammu and Kashmir

- Ms Nasira Parvin (Lady Health Visitor Supervisor)
- Ms Khalida Parvin (Lady Health Visitor Supervisor)
- Dr Zahid Chatta (Programme Manager, Basic Development Needs Programme)

Experts who were consulted to clarify administrative and technical issues and who consented to disclose their names and identities

- Dr Zubair Hasan MBBS, MCPS, MPH (Public Health Scientist/Hospital Manager)
- Dr Shahzad Ali Khan MBBS, MBA, MPH, PhD, FRSPH (Researcher/Teacher/University Level/Assistant Professor)
- Mr Qamar-ul-Islam Siddiqui MS (Sociology), MPH (International Health) (Public Health Communication Specialist)

Nongovernmental organizations/community-based organizations that coordinated with the researcher in organizing interviews and focus group discussions in the four selected districts

- Muslim Welfare Society, Hyderabad, Sindh
- Basic Development Needs Programme, Jamshoro, Sindh
- Bunyad, Lahore, Punjab
- Basic Development Needs Programme, Kasur, Punjab
- Kohsar, Muzaffarabad, Azad Jammu and Kashmir
- Basic Development Needs Programme, Muzaffarabad, Azad Jammu and Kashmir

Annex 3. General profiles of the districts included in the study

Sindh

Hyderabad is the second largest city in Sindh province and is the sixth largest city in the country. Hyderabad is where the district headquarters are located and the district government is seated.

Administrative divisions

Before the Government of Zulfiqar Ali Bhutto, Hyderabad district was included in the present-day district of Badin. Then in the 1990s it was again divided into four more districts: Matairi, Tando Allahyar, Tando Mohammad Khan and the present-day Hyderabad district. The Hyderabad district was again subdivided into four talukas, which are the smallest districts of Sindh province: Hyderabad City, Hyderabad Rural, Latifabad and Qasimabad.

Demographics

Hyderabad is noteworthy in Sindh, and in Pakistan generally, for its relative tolerance towards religious and ethnic affairs. During independence of Pakistan in 1947, a large number of Muslim refugees escaped from the programmes and genocide in India and settled in Hyderabad. Today, native Sindhi- and non-Sindhi speaking Sindhis live in harmony after a brief history of conflict. A large influx of Pashtuns and Punjabis were attracted to Hyderabad after the Indus treaty settlement. Most Punjabis mixed with the local population; however, most Pashtuns remained distinct and lived separately. The city therefore has a cosmopolitan atmosphere, with multiethnic and multicultural communities.

Hindus account for the largest religious minority, forming 12% of the total population of the city. Although Christians account for just 4% of the total population, Hyderabad is the seat of a Diocese of the Church of Pakistan and has five churches and a cathedral. Despite its strategic location and thrifty people, the city is under the shadow of Karachi and has yet to make its mark economically. One reason for this is the artificial factional and sectarian isolation imposed after the riots of the late 1980s and early 1990s, which divided the urban population.

Jamshoro is a city in Jamshoro district, Sindh. It is located on the right bank of the Indus river, approximately 18 km north-west of the city of Hyderabad and 150 km north-east of the provincial capital Karachi. It is the gateway to the Indus valley, world famous for its civilization and rich cultural heritage.

Dadu is a district of Sindh. Dadu district was created in 1933 by the British Indian administration who merged Kotri and Kohistan tehsils from Karachi district and Mehar, Khairpur Nathan Shah, Dadu, Johi and Sehwan tehsils from Larkana district. According to 1998 census report, the population of the district is 1 688 810. The district constitutes 79% and 21% of the total rural and urban population, respectively. It has an area of 19 070 km^2 divided into seven talukas, yielding a population density of 88.6 persons/km^2. The average household size in the district is 5.5 persons (6.3 in urban areas and 5.3 in rural areas). More than 73% of the housing units in

Dadu district are single room houses. The average annual rainfall in the district is about 120 mm. The total area under forest is 217 000 ha, yielding timber and firewood. In 2004, another district by the name of Jamshoro was carved out of Dadu district, which comprised Kotri taluka, Sehwan taluka and Jamshoro taluka, which is the headquarters of the new district.

The demographic indicators of the district at the 1998 census (including Jamshoro district, which was a part of Dadu at that time) showed that 97.49% of the population were Muslim, 2.05% were Hindu, 0.37% were Christian, 0.08% were Ahmadiyya Muslims and 0.02% followed other religions. Hindus and Christians are mainly concentrated in urban areas.

Languages

The following languages are spoken: Sindhi (50.0%), Seraiki (43.33%), Urdu (2.56%), Punjabi (1.88%), Pashto (1.17%), Baluchi (0.42%) and others (0.28%).

Urdu speakers are mainly concentrated in urban areas.

Punjab

Kasur

Kasur district is one of the districts in the province of Punjab. It came into existence on 1 July 1976; earlier it was part of Lahore district. The district capital is Kasur city. The total area of the district is 3995 km^2. According to the 1998 census, the total population of the district is 2 376 000. Of this, 95.4% are Muslim, 4.4% are Christian while the remainder are Ahmadis, Hindus and scheduled castes. A total of 22.78% live in urban areas. The district is administratively subdivided into four tehsils and 141 union councils: Chunian (27 union councils), Kasur (55 union councils), Pattoki (31 union councils) and Kot Radha Kishen (28 union councils).

Azad Jammu and Kashmir

Muzaffarabad is the capital of Azad Jammu and Kashmir. It is located in Muzaffarabad district on the banks of the Jhelum and Neelum rivers. The district is bounded by Khyber-Pakhtunkhwa in the west, by the Kupwara and Baramulla districts on the Indian side of the Line of Control in the east, and the Neelum district of Azad Jammu and Kashmir in the north. According to the 1998 census, the population of the district was 725 000, and according to a 1999 projection, the population had risen to almost 741 000. The district comprises three tehsils, and the city of Muzaffarabad serves as the capital of Azad Jammu and Kashmir.

Health profiles of the districts included in the study

Muzaffarabad district, Azad Jammu and Kashmir

Population	700 000
Hospitals	2 (Abbas Institute of Medical Sciences and a combined military hospital)
Tehsil headquarters	2
Rural health centres	4
Basic health units	47
Medical officers	44 (excluding two big hospitals)
Lady health visitors	65 (excluding two big hospitals)
Lady health workers	655

Kasur district, Punjab

Population	2 375 875
District headquarters	1
Tehsil headquarters	2
Rural health centres	12
Basic health units	81

Hyderabad district, Sindh

Population	1 847 106
Total health facilities	55
Vaccinators	137
Expanded Programme on Immunization centres	60
Lady health visitors	43
Lady health workers	1184

Annex 4. Profiles of the health service providers in the four districts

Table 1. Profile of the health service providers in Hyderabad district.

Health service provider	No. of years of service	Training received on gender	Training received on gender-based violence	Training received on gender and health issues	Training received on health issues
Lady health workers	6	No	No	Yes	Yes
Lady health visitors	2	No	No	No	Yes
Medical officers (female)	10	No	No	No	Yes
Medical officers (male)	28	Yes	Yes	Yes	Yes
Executive district officers/district health officers	30	No	No	No	Yes

Table 2. Profile of the health service providers in Jamshoro district.

Health service provider	No. of years of service	Training received on gender	Training received on gender-based violence	Training received on gender and health issues	Training received on health issues
Lady health workers	3	No	No	Yes (6)	Yes/many
Lady health visitors	10	No	No	No	Yes/many
Medical officers (female)	10	Yes	No	No	Yes/many
Medical officers (male)	15	Yes	No	No	Yes/many
Tehsil health officers[a]	15	Yes	No	No	Yes/many

[a]Executive district officers – data not available.

Table 3. Profile of the health service providers in Muzaffarabad district.

Health service provider	No. of years of service	Training received on gender	Training received on gender-based violence	Training received on gender and health issues	Training received on health issues
Lady health workers	9	No	No	No	No
Lady health visitors	12	No	No	No	Yes (5)
Medical officers (female)	6	Yes (2)	No	Yes (1)	Yes (7)
Medical officers (male)	5	Yes (2)	No	Yes (1)	Yes (6)
District health officers	25	No	No	No	Yes

Table 4. Profile of the health service providers in Kasur district.

Health service provider	No. of years of service	Training received on gender	Training received on gender-based violence	Training received on gender and health issues	Training received on health issues
Lady health workers	8	No	No	Yes	Yes
Lady health visitors	15	No	No	Yes	Yes
Medical officers (female)	3	No	No	Yes	Yes
Medical officers (male)	15	No	No	Yes	Yes
Executive district officers/district health officers	25	No	No	Yes	Yes

Table 5. A quantified summary of the understanding of gender, gender-based violence and related issues by the health service providers in the four districts.[62]

Issue	Districts																			
	Hyderabad					Jamshoro					Muzaffarabad					Kasur				
Health service provider responses	LHWs	LHVs	MOs (F)	MOs (M)	HOs	LHWs	LHVs	MOs (F)	MOs (M)	HOs	LHWs	LHVs	MOs (F)	MOs (M)	HOs	LHWs	LHVs	MOs (F)	MOs (M)	HOs
Familiarity with the word "gender/*sinf*"	Yes	Yes	Yes	Yes	Yes	Yes	Yes	Yes	Yes	Yes	Yes	Yes	Yes	Yes	Yes	Yes	Yes	Yes	Yes	Yes
Understanding of the difference between sex and gender	Yes	Yes	Yes	Yes	Yes	Yes	Yes	Yes	Yes	Yes	Yes	Yes	Yes	Yes	Yes	Yes	Yes	Yes	Yes	Yes
Violence exists in lives of Pakistani women	Yes	Yes	Yes	Yes	Yes	Yes	Yes	Yes	Yes		Yes	Yes	Yes	Yes	Yes	Yes	Yes	Yes	Yes	Yes
Violence is in the lives of women in their district	Yes	Yes	Yes	Yes	Yes	Yes	Yes	Yes	Yes	Yes	Yes	Yes	Yes	Yes	Yes	Yes	Yes	Yes	Yes	Yes
Gender-based violence/violence against women is a public health issue	Yes	Yes	Yes	Yes	Yes	Yes	Yes	Yes	Yes	Yes	Yes	Yes	Yes	Yes	Yes	Yes	Yes	Yes	Yes	Yes

F, female; HOs, health officers (executive district officers or district health officers); LHVs, lady health visitors; LHWs, lady health workers; M, male; MOs, medical officers.

[62] Most of the health service providers have heard the word "gender". However, most could not differentiate between sex and gender at the conceptual level. Among lady health visitors and lady health workers, all those who had the chance of any health session in connection with family and rural health programmes or those who had attended a two-day workshop by WHO in 2010, knew about the word "gender/*sinf*". Table 5 needs to be carefully evaluated and understood. One could be mislead by seeing all the "Yes" responses. An in-depth session clarified the exact level of understanding and perception. Some know that it is "nice and wise" to admit that gender-based violence is a public health issue but "in fact there is no such relation" or "what can health service providers do for violence against women?". Therefore, for all practical purposes, policy-makers and donors should aim towards integrating gender-based violence in the health sector from a beginner's level.

Annex 5. Profiles of the respondents of the focus group discussions

Table 1. Profile of the urban male respondents, Hyderabad district, Sindh.

Parameter	Respondent						
	1	2	3	4	5	6	7
Age (years)	29	26	29	32	47	30	27
Education	BA	Intermediate	Bachelor of Arts	Bachelor of Arts	Master of Arts	Nil	Nil
Marital status	Married	Single	Married	Married	Married	Married	Married
No. of children	2	0	2	1	5	3	2
Employment status	Private	Private	Private	Government	Government	Private	Private
Access to television	Yes	Yes	Yes	Yes	Yes	Yes	Yes
Access to mobile phone	Yes	Yes	Yes	Yes	Yes	Yes	Yes
Access to radio	Yes	Yes	Yes	Yes	Yes	Yes	Yes
Access to newspaper	Yes	Yes	Yes	Yes	Yes	Yes	yes
Any disability	No	No	No	No	No	No	No

Table 2. Profile of the urban male respondents, Jamshoro district, Sindh.

Parameter	Respondent					
	1	2	3	4	5	6
Age (years)	29	35	38	28	27	21
Education	Intermediate	Bachelor of Arts	Bachelor of Arts	Bachelor of Arts	Matriculated	Intermediate
Marital status	Married	Married	Married	–	Married	–
No. of children	2	1	3	0	2	0
Employment status	Business	Government	Shopkeeper	–	Labourer	–
Access to television	Yes	Yes	Yes	Yes	Yes	Yes
Access to mobile phone	Yes	Yes	Yes	Yes	Yes	Yes
Access to radio	Yes	Yes	Yes	Yes	Yes	Yes
Access to newspaper	Yes	Yes	Yes	Yes	Yes	Yes
Any disability	No	No	No	No	No	No

Table 3. Profile of the urban male respondents, Muzaffarabad district, Azad Jammu and Kashmir.

es".meter	Respondent				
	1	2	3	4	5
Age (years)	35	32	29	32	40
Education	Matriculated	Master of Arts	Middle	Bachelor of Arts	Middle
Marital status	Married	Married	Married	Married	Married
No. of children	2	2	1	2	3
Employment status	Labourer/daily wages	Government service	Driver	Journalist	Teacher
Access to television	Yes	Yes	Yes	Yes	Yes
Access to mobile phone	Yes	Yes	Yes	Yes	Yes
Access to radio	Yes	Yes	Yes	Yes	Yes
Access to newspaper	Yes	Yes	Yes	Yes	Yes
Any disability	No	No	No	No	No

Table 4. Profile of the semi-urban male respondents, Kasur district, Punjab.

Parameter	Respondent							
	1	2	3	4	5	6	7	8
Age (years)	32	46	42	39	51	27	40	34
Education	Matriculated	Middle	Illiterate	Primary	Illiterate	Bachelor of Arts, Bachelor of Education	Illiterate	Faculty of Arts
Marital status	Single	Married	Married	Married	Married	Single	Married	Married
No. of children	0	3	4	3	7	0	5	2
Employment status	Unemployed	Factory worker	Rickshaw driver	Labourer	Farmer	School teacher	Farmer	Private
Access to television	Yes	Yes	Yes	Yes	Yes	Yes	Yes	Yes
Access to mobile phone	Yes	Yes	Yes	Yes	Yes	Yes	Yes	Yes
Access to radio	No	No	Yes	No	Yes	No	Yes	No
Access to newspaper	Yes	No	No	No	No	Yes	No	Yes
Any disability	No	No	No	No	No	No	No	No

Table 5. Profile of the urban female respondents, Hyderabad district, Sindh.

Parameter	Respondent					
	1	2	3	4	5	6
Age (years)	40	30	29	22	27	33
Education/no. of years of schooling	10	12	12	12	10	5
Marital status	Married	Married	Married	Single	Not disclosed	Married
No. of children	4	1	2	0	0	3
Employment status	Housewife	Housewife	Domestic worker	–	Housewife	Domestic worker
Access to television	Yes	Yes	Yes	Yes	Yes	Yes
Access to mobile phone	Yes	Yes	Yes	Yes	Yes	Yes
Access to radio	Yes	Yes	Yes	Yes	Yes	Yes
Access to newspaper	Yes	Yes	Yes	Yes	Yes	Yes
Any disability	No	No	No	No	No	No
Any other attribute	No	No	No	No	No	No
Purdah observing/veiled	Yes	Yes	Yes	No	Yes	No

Table 6. Profile of the urban female respondents, Jamshoro district, Sindh.

Parameter	Respondent					
	1	2	3	4	5	6
Age (years)	28	38	29	30	39	35
Education	–	–	–	–	Matriculated	Primary
Marital status	Married	Married	Married	Married	Married	Married
No. of children	1	3	3	2	4	5
Employment status	Housewife	Housewife	Housewife	Housewife	Housewife	Housewife
Access to television	Yes	Yes	Yes	Yes	Yes	Yes
Access to mobile phone	Yes	No	No	Yes	Yes	Yes
Access to radio	Yes	Yes	Yes	Yes	Yes	Yes
Access to newspaper	Yes	Yes	Yes	Yes	Yes	Yes
Any disability	No	No	No	No	No	No
Purdah observing/veiled	Yes	Yes	Yes	Yes	No	No

Table 7. Profile of the urban female respondents, Muzaffarabad district, Azad Jammu and Kashmir.

Parameter	Respondent							
	1	2	3	4	5	6	7	8
Age (years)	21	24	29	37	39	32	28	41
Education	Faculty of Arts	Bachelor of Arts	Middle	Illiterate	Primary	Illiterate	Matriculated	Middle
Marital status	Married	Married	Married	Married	Married	Married	–	Married
No. of children	1	2	1	5	3	3	0	6
Employment status	Housewife	Housewife	Housewife	Housewife	Housewife	Housewife	Housewife	Housewife
Access to television	Yes	Yes	Yes	Yes	Yes	Yes	Yes	Yes
Access to mobile phone	Yes	Yes	Yes	Yes	Yes	Yes	Yes	Yes
Access to radio	Yes	Yes	Yes	Yes	Yes	Yes	Yes	Yes
Access to newspaper	Yes	Yes	Yes	Yes	Yes	YES	Yes	Yes
Any disability	No	No	No	No	No	No	No	No
Purdah observing/veiled	Yes	No	Yes	Yes	No	No	No	No

Table 8. Profile of the semi-urban female respondents, Kasur district, Punjab.

Parameter	Respondent							
	1	2	3	4	5	6	7	8
Age (years)	44	48	39	53	23	52	49	38
Education	Illiterate	Illiterate	Primary	Illiterate	Bachelor of Arts	Illiterate	Primary	Illiterate
Marital status	Married	Married	Married	Married	Single	Married	Married	Married
No. of children	5	6	4	7	0	6	2	3
Employment status	Housewife	Housewife	Housewife	Housewife	Student	Housewife	Housewife	Housewife
Access to television	Yes	Yes	Yes	Yes	Yes	Yes	Yes	Yes
Access to mobile phone	Yes	Yes	Yes	Yes	Yes	No	No	Yes
Access to radio	No	No	No	No	No	No	Yes	No
Access to newspaper	No	No	No	No	Yes	No	No	No
Any disability	No	No	No	No	No	No	No	No
Purdah observing/veiled	No	No	No	No	No	No	No	No

References

Bott S & Betron M (2005). *USAID-funded gender-based violence programming: An assessment report for the Bureau of Child Health*. Washington DC, United States Agency for International Development.

Bott S, Morrison A & Ellsberg M (2005). *Preventing and responding to gender-based violence in middle and low-income countries: A global review and analysis*. Washington DC, World Bank.

BRAC (2003). *An assessment of male attitude towards violence against women*. Dhaka, BRAC (http://www.bracresearch.org/others/an_assessment_of_male_attitude_towards_violence_against_women_pdf.pdf, accessed November 2010).

Burney S (1999). *Crime or custom? Violence against women in Pakistan*. Pakistan, Human Rights Watch (http://www.unhcr.org/refworld/docid/45d314242.html, accessed November 2011).

Human Rights Watch (1996) *The Human Rights Watch global report on women's human rights*. New York, Human Rights Watch (http://www.wwda.org.au/hrwgolbalrept1.pdf, accessed November 2010).

Commonwealth of Australia (2008). *Addressing violence against women in Melanesia and East Timor: Solomon Islands country supplement*. Canberra, Office of Development Effectiveness.

DoH (2005). *Responding to domestic abuse: A handbook for health professionals*. United Kingdom, Department of Health (http://www.dh.gov.uk/prod_consum_dh/groups/dh_digitalassets/@dh/@en/documents/digitalasset/dh_4126619.pdf, accessed November 2010).

Du Mont J & White D (2008). *Global review of the role of medico-legal evidence in sexual assault cases*. Sexual Violence Research initiative (http://www.svri.org/WHOSVRIGlobalMedicolegalReview.pdf, accessed November 2010).

Garcia-Moreno C (2005). *Violence against women worldwide*. New York, United Nations Development Fund for Women (http://www.unifem.org/campaigns/sayno/docs/SayNOunite_FactSheet_VAWworldwide.pdf, accessed November 2010)

Guedes A (2004) *Addressing gender-based violence from the reproductive health/HIV sector: A lierature review and analysis*. POPTECH Publication Number 04-164-020. Washington DC, Interagency Working Group (www.prb.org/pdf04/addressGendrBasedViolence.pdf, accessed November 2010).

Hausmann R, Tyson LD & Zahidi S (2009). *The global gender gap report, 2009*. Geneva, World Economic Forum (http://members.weforum.org/pdf/gendergap/report2009.pdf, accessed November 2010).

Hausmann R, Tyson LD & Zahidi S (2010). *The global gender gap report, 2010*. Geneva, World Economic Forum (http://www3.weforum.org/docs/WEF_GenderGap_Report_2010.pdf, accessed November 2010).

Heise L, Ellsberg M & Gottemoeller M (1999). *Ending violence against women*. Population Reports: Volume XXVII, Number 4, Series L, Number 11, Issues in World Health (http://info.k4health.org/pr/l11/violence.pdf, accessed November 2010).

IntraHealth International (2008). *Twubakane GBV/PMTCT readiness assessment toolkit*. Chapel Hill, North Carolina, IntraHealth International.

Jewkes R & Morrell R (2010). Gender and sexuality: emerging perspectives from the heterosexual epidemic in South Africa and implications for HIV risk and prevention. *Journal of the International AIDS Society*, 13(1):6.

Morgan P (1997). *The design and use of capacity development indicators*. Paper prepared for the Policy Branch of the Canadian International Development Agency (http://www.mekonginfo.org/HDP/Lib.nsf/0/18A3C57E35F91A9E47256D80002F7C81/$FILE/CIDA%20-%20Capacity%20Development%20Indicators%201997.PDF, accessed November 2010).

Perveen R (2010). *Violence against women in Pakistan: A qualitative review of statistics for 2009. Annual Report Jan–Dec 2009*. Policy and Data Monitoring on Violence Against Women Project, in collaboration with the Violence against Women Watch group and supported by TroCaire. Islamabad, Aurat Foundation.

UN (2006). *In-depth study on all forms of violence against women: Report of the Secretary General*. Geneva, United Nations General Assembly.

UNDP (2010). *Human development report 2010 – 20th anniversary edition. The real wealth of nations: Pathways to human development*. Geneva, United Nations Population Fund (http://hdr.undp.org/en/reports/global/hdr2010, accessed November 2010).

UNFPA (2001). *A practical approach to gender-based violence: A program guide for health care providers and managers*. New York, United Nations Population Fund.

UNFPA (2010). *Health sector response to gender-based violence: An assessment of the Asia Pacific Region*. Bangkok, United Nations Population Fund, Asia and the Pacific Office.

USAID (2008). *Addressing gender-based violence through USAID's program: A guide for health sector program officers*. Washington DC, United States Agency for International Development.

WHO (2002). *World report on violence and health*. Geneva, World Health Organization.

WHO (2005). *Multi-country study on women's health and domestic violence against women: Initial results on prevalence, health outcomes and women's responses*. Geneva, World Health Organization.

WUNRN (2004). *Glossary of violence against women. Committee on the status of women (nongovernmental organization working group on violence against women)*. Women's United Nations Report Network (http://www.wunrn.com/reference/pdf/glossary_vaw.pdf, accessed November 2010).